Advance Praise for
The Gentle Art of Newborn Family Care

Salle Webber's beautiful book, The Gentle Art of Newborn Family Care, *weaves ancient wisdom with practical guidance. Salle's poetic writing inspires and nourishes the reader, whether a doula, family caregiver, new mother or father. She illuminates the importance of tending mother-baby couplets with great care during their most profound beginnings. Her insight gifts us with secure babies, confident mothers, and healthy families as she shares her expertise with sensitivity, humor, and grace.*
—Maggie Muir, MA, LMFT, Family Wellness for the Childbearing Years, Soquel, CA

I loved the warm feeling I was left with after reading the book. It does a great job of relaying the important of parent-to-parent support during breastfeeding. I wish this amazing resource was available before my wife and I had our first.
—Scott Sherwood, Executive Director, U.S. Lactation Consultant Association

In The Gentle Art of Newborn Family Care, *Salle Webber describes simply and eloquently what every doula (and grandparent!) needs to know to be of genuine help to new families. In doing so, she also conveys the essential elements of true support,   such as putting the parents' priorities above your own. Webber brings an open mind and heart to the families she serves, and her book models the attitudes those who work with new families—including breastfeeding supporters—would be wise to cultivate. She describes some of the lessons and attitudes that took me decades to figure out. It's a profound work that I hope will have a great impact.*
—Nancy Mohrbacher, IBCLC, FILCA, author *Breastfeeding Answers Made Simple* and co-author of *Breastfeeding Made Simple: Seven Natural Laws for Nursing Mothers*

This gem of a book reflects Salle Webber's experience as a mother and as a postpartum doula for the past 25 years. Written to "help us care for one another," Webber provides a heart-centered model for the kind of assistance needed to get families, in all kinds of situations, off to the best possible start.
—Marian Tompson, Founder, La Leche League International, author, *Passionate Journey: My Unexpected Life*

Salle's book is a wonderfully gentle guide about how to help the new mother and the newborn during their babymoon. She discusses all the facets of the postpartum doula role. The depth of her experience as a "grandmother for hire" is obvious in every chapter. Her understanding of the emotional and physical needs of the mother, the newborn baby, and the emergent family as a whole is beautiful in breadth and depth. I love the overall emotional tone of this book. I could feel the author's genuine gentle, loving, and accepting wisdom... What a wonderful gift to bring to the conversation our society is having about new moms, newborn babies, and emergent families! She has written an accessible book that explains and provides practical supportive solutions, based in love and acceptance, regarding the needs of the new mother, newborn care, and the emergent family. Her life's work as a postpartum doula is good work, work that directly affects new families.
—Kathy Morelli, LPC, Marriage and Family Counselor, author of *BirthTouch®: Shiatsu and Acupressure for the Childbearing Year*

Reading Salle's book, The Gentle Art of Newborn Family Care, *is like listening to a favorite aunt tell stories about the babies she has helped and the mothers that she nurtured. Salle has captured the essence of postpartum doula care in her guidance and support of the new mother, and her encouragement to know the baby and especially how to soothe a newborn (with the goal of education and equipping the parents with this knowledge). I just read this book over a weekend while teaching a doula training, and it was such a great overview that I think this book should be added to the reading lists of all the doula training organizations as a modern representation of the heart and work of the postpartum doula. Written in an easy format for those beginning doula care, or families who might be interested in what a doula does; this book was also rich for me to read (as a full-time doula of a dozen years). Reading along makes you want to invite Salle into your home, or find a doula who is a lot like her! What a great representation of our calling as non-judgmental support, nurturing education, and knowledge of resources to recommend. A treasure for the postpartum doula community.*
—Kimberly Bepler, IBCLC, CPD/CPDT, ICPE, CST, ABC Doula Service

The Gentle Art of Newborn and Family Care *by Salle Webber is a must read for all postpartum doulas and those considering this profession. The warm touch, the honest look at the life inside the heart and business of a postpartum doula is quite unique. The rich details of the everyday and seemingly mundane tasks that help a postpartum family unite are treated with deserving respect, though Webber doesn't mince words about the business aspects either. I really liked this book! There isn't anything like it on the market. I'm excited to be able to send people to it when I'm asked for a guide.*

—Robin Elise Weiss, MPH, CPH, CD(DONA), BDT(DONA),
ICPFE, CLC, LCCE, FACCE

The Gentle Art of Newborn Family Care

A Guide for Doulas and Caregivers

Salle Webber

To Carol,
You were one of my
earliest mothering-models,
and such an inspiration!
With love + Gratitude,
Salle ♡

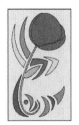

Praeclarus Press, LLC

www.PraeclarusPress.com

Praeclarus Press, LLC
2504 Sweetgum Lane
Amarillo, Texas 79124 USA
806-367-9950
www.PraeclarusPress.com

DISCLAIMER

The information contained in this publication is advisory only and is not intended to replace sound clinical judgment or individualized patient care. The author disclaims all warranties, whether expressed or implied, including any warranty as the quality, accuracy, safety, or suitability of this information for any particular purpose.

ISBN: 978-0-9854180-0-7
ISBN (Kindle): 978-0-9854180-2-1
ISBN (Nook): 978-0-9854180-5-2

Cover Design: Ken Tackett

Front Cover Photo: Maggie Muir

Back Cover Photo: Jeane Michioka

Developmental Editing: Kathleen Kendall-Tackett

Copy Editing: Diana Cassar-Uhl

Layout & Design: Todd Rollison

Illustration: Ken Tackett

Doula Logo Design: Lawrence Hansen

Table of Contents

SECTION II: THE SKILLS OF CARE

FOREWORD

As I read through the manuscript of Salle Webber's book, I was struck by how much, as a young mother many years ago, I would have cherished her gentle open-hearted guidance and wisdom after each of my four babies was born. This hit home especially when I read her words, "My bottom-line day-to-day philosophy of the work of a doula is to meet the needs of the mother . . . ." With the dishes piled in the sink, a mountain of laundry accumulating, a sore bottom, and a baby crying while a toddler needed something to eat, I often felt overwhelmed, incompetent, exhausted and upset with myself, but also defensive when my mother-in-law commented on the mess. I needed a Salle many times. I still recall that desperation and loneliness, even though that was a half century ago. I tried to make sure that when my children grew up and had new babies, they would get the best care that I and the "other grandmother" could give. We could have used Salle's book for those eight grandchildren!

Now we have the postpartum doula. Salle is one of the originals, a self-made doula, a "natural" if there ever was one. As a young mother herself, she recognized the needs of new parents and felt an affinity for them as well as a love and understanding of tiny babies. By now, she has worked with all sorts of babies and parents–healthy term babies, twins, adopted babies, preterm and sick babies, breastfed and formula-fed babies. She has worked with single and partnered mothers, old and young, first-time and experienced mothers. Her good instincts and natural humility won the hearts of the parents she served, and she has changed lives as a result. She models the need for flexibility and acceptance of the values and lifestyle of the families she serves.

With this book she shares lots and lots of practical tips, sprinkled with wisdom and guidance. Her conversational tone, numerous stories and examples, and heartwarming photos make this a very good read for other doulas, parents and those loved ones and friends who want to help new parents.

One of the most important lessons from Salle (besides, "Be sure you know how to soothe a crying baby!") is this: "The advantage of the doula is that she has no agenda other than service, no need to push her opinions, and no complex history with either parent that can cloud the moment." For those of us who work with childbearing families, caring for people whose values are different from our own can be challenging. Sometimes our way of dealing with such differences is to try to change their attitudes and behavior. An uneasy and awkward relationship results, and too often, the new parents feel judged and reluctant to change. Furthermore, they may feel "stuck" because of a contract or prepayment for services. Both parties are dissatisfied. We should take Salle's words very seriously, even though at times, this is easier said than done.

I feel our role as doulas is to take on the values of our clients as our own, for the duration of the relationship. We are like chameleons, changing our colors, depending on the environment. It really helps to discover the basis of her values, preferences, and behavior. Knowing this gives us a context for understanding. Usually, through conversation, good listening, and observation, we can gain that understanding. The bottom line is that if we don't agree with her and do not know why she feels and acts as she does, we must tell ourselves that she has very good reasons for her values, decisions, and behavior. This will help us be supportive and not judgmental. Once trust and respect are established, mothers and others are more open to suggestions that may help solve common problems in mothers' recovery and in infant care and feeding.

Salle personifies this attitude consistently in her stories and her advice, thus showing the benefits to all of accepting the family's values.

Enjoy and learn from this wise, compassionate and humble expert, who has launched hundreds of newborn families over her 25-year career. Using her guidance you can multiply the goodness many times over, and the families you serve will be most grateful.

Penny Simkin

—Penny Simkin, PT, is a childbirth educator, birth doula, birth counselor, and author or co-author of many books and articles for parents and professionals including, The Birth Partner: A Guide for Dads, Doulas, and All Other Labor Companions. *She is a Founder of DONA International. (www.pennysimkin.com)*

ACKNOWLEDGEMENTS

This work gestated for years before it was ready to be born into the world. It has taken the support of my village to guide it into life. I have so many people to thank.

- To every family who opened their lives to me in their time of tender transition, I am grateful. The hours I spent in each home are the stuff of which this book is written. It would not exist without you.

- To Laura Davis and the original Friday morning feedback group, thank you for guiding me to find the voice within me that could be heard. Thanks for all the listening, caring, and honing of sentences. My treasured writing buddy Karen Rowe has nurtured my work through all phases of its process.

- To my friend Stacey Dennick, who has encouraged, inspired, and teased me into keeping up the writing, offering an editorial eye and a place to write. I lovingly thank you.

- To Liz Koch, ahead-of-her-time founder of *The Doula* magazine, who gave a name to my work. Carrying the magazine on was Michele Winkler, to whom I give thanks for the gentle prodding to write the piece that ultimately connected me with my publisher.

- To April Stearns, my former student, thanks for your belief in this project. I look forward to reading your book one day. To Fern, Michael, and Kapoli, my Kaua'i family, *aloha pumehana* for the ongoing hospitality and friendship without which I could never have accomplished this. You are always in my heart.

- To Maggie Muir, my undying gratitude for your continual support of this book's goals and vision, your editorial assistance, wonderful photographs, and your belief in me and the work we do. The incredible Santa Cruz birthing community has been a marvelous source of peer support and inspiration. You know who you are! And to Jill Esteras, my friend and former neighbor who so clearly pointed out my life's work, thank you for noticing.

- To everyone who offered their photos for use on these pages, I appreciate your willingness to share your tender moments with the world. They bring a sense of truth and reality to the words.

- To my family: my husband Leo, my children Noel, Lilia, and Aerielle, and my beloved grandchildren, you are the ones who truly gave me the training in motherhood that brought me to where I am and what I do. My love for being a mother to a growing family is what led me to this work.

- And of course to Kathy Kendall-Tackett, my publisher and editor, you carried the torch for many years unknown to me, but we are a match made in heaven. I am so glad we finally found each other! May our offspring...this text...thrive and grow, serve and illuminate, adding momentum to the movement toward gentle beginnings.

PREFACE

Giving birth in the twenty-first century is a complex experience. Though every human on Earth arrived through the body of its mother, the simplicity of natural birth has been replaced with routine hospital technology. Bringing the baby home, parents are faced with continuing dilemmas of social expectations and the latest baby-training fad. They are not encouraged to listen to their own inner knowing or to trust themselves to care for their child. There is an expert at every turn waiting to advise on the right or wrong way to raise a baby. The importance of simple things—like feeding the infant—is often overlooked, while the consumption-of-goods factor is magnified.

Parents may find that some of these ideas may have merit, while others seem to require going against the wisdom of their hearts. They may be uncomfortable using formula, though the doctor said it was all the same, or letting their baby cry when they feel she just wants to be held. They don't want to supplement with a bottle, they want to work to get their milk production up. That cute outfit seems so uncomfortable, though everyone is complementing it. Why is the baby squirmy and fussy? The stroller is nice, but maybe for when the baby is older. For now, a mother may prefer to carry or wrap her child against her body. Perhaps a new mom is not inclined to take her baby out right away, but is feeling pressure to rejoin activities and gatherings. These and many other contradictions come up for new parents today, and they need support in maintaining what is innately best for themselves and their newborn child.

It will be some time before the mother-and-baby couple is ready to introduce themselves to the community outside the home. They need to gain physical strength and endurance, the mother replenishing her body that carried and delivered a child, and the infant establishing his connection to Earth and humanity, learning to feed well, sleep, and grow.

Our culture is without a custom that provides for the care and well-being of this new family as they progress. The mother may exist for weeks in a blur of sleep deprivation, lack of companionship, insufficient food or drink throughout the day, limited ability to attend to her personal hygiene needs, confusing demands from the baby, and in some cases, depression as a result. The outside world is going on without her. Her partner is back to work after a week or two at most; her friends are busy and seem so well-dressed when they drop in. Her clothes don't fit, her breasts are enormous and dripping milk. She hasn't had a conversation with an adult in hours—or days. Her focus is on putting the baby to her breast, milk let-down, burping, pooping, and spitting up. The modern world is less than interested, and she may feel isolated and alone.

One caring person can change all that. Daily attention and companionship are therapeutic. Sharing the wonder of the child is a lovely experience for all. Remember the miracle that this new life represents, and know that it is an honor to be part of this circle.

We are learning once again how to attend to the needs of our neighbors. Bringing food, cleaning house, entertaining older children, or simply listening and encouraging are simple yet vital services we can offer. Looking with compassion upon a tired mother, we may offer to hold the baby while she naps, or to do the laundry, or prepare dinner, go grocery shopping, or massage her weary back. These are the simple necessities so often overlooked.

Modern society is based on facts, on science, making it no wonder that the art of newborn family care has become one of the lost arts of our time. It is far too fluid and emotion-based, too watery, and unpredictable; illogical, certainly. New mothers cannot be expected to live by the usual rules of society. They require care that meets the needs of the partnership they share with their babies. As we better understand the importance of the early weeks of life to the child's later expectations and behaviors, we see the value in being compassionate. As we reflect on the long-term health benefits, physical as well as mental, of full healing after a major medical event, we see the importance of caring for our new mothers.

MY STORY

I birthed my first child at age 24. Typical of my generation, I knew next to nothing about birth or babies, but I was confident that it would come naturally. I took a Lamaze class in preparation for birth, and was clear with my doctor that I wanted no intervention or drugs. The year was 1972. Breastfeeding was coming back after several decades of "expert advice" that infant formula was the best food for babies. I was certain I would breastfeed, and fortunately, it came easily to my son and me, as there was no one to assist us.

Noel's birth was normal and unmedicated, though my pubic hairs were shaved and my bag of waters broken immediately upon checking in to the hospital, to "move things along faster." It was standard procedure to keep mother and child hospitalized for four days after a normal birth.

Immediately after he was born, my son was taken from me for 12 hours of observation: the longest 12 hours of my life. I was advised to rest, but I was filled with energy from the birth and wanted desperately to hold my baby. It felt so wrong … my womb was empty, but so were my arms. Finally we were reunited, and I put him to my breast. His mouth was eager, and it was all so new. I was excited to explore his little energetic body, to kiss and smell him, to soothe and caress him. But too soon, the nurse came to take him away; she was clearly in charge of my son. From then on, Noel was kept in a nursery, and brought to me every four hours, regardless of his cries for food or comfort. I felt powerless and empty. My baby and I needed each other, and regulations kept us apart. The needs of breastfeeding infants were not understood at that time. A formula-fed child can go four hours without eating, but breast milk, and its forerunner, colostrum, are so easily digested and assimilated, the newborn needs to feed more frequently.

Finally, we were released from the hospital. Going home was a relief. At last I would be allowed to attend to my baby, hold him as much as he needed, feed him when he was hungry rather than when the clock, or the nurses, said to. I found that he would cry the moment I'd put him down. Even if he fell asleep at my breast, putting him in his cradle woke him. I felt sure that he had become fearful of losing me, from the painful routine of separation during his first days of life. His father was helpful, but it was me the baby wanted, and I surrendered to being constantly available to him.

We were living with my brother and his girlfriend. She had a two-year-old son. She was a teenage mom and a voracious reader. She offered me no assistance when I came home from the hospital, didn't prepare meals, or take over chores. I remember watching her, engrossed in her reading, as I struggled to tend to my baby and keep the whole family fed and cared for. She wasn't cruel, just young, oblivious, and self-centered.

I was exhausted, but committed to my baby's well-being. My mother-model was my good friend Carol, who had birthed her son a year earlier. I observed her style of mothering, which was naturally fluid and responsive. She held her son and nursed him whenever he desired. She took him with her everywhere. He was a beautiful, contented child. To this day I am grateful to Carol for showing me the way.

Noel was difficult to satisfy. My feeling of being overwhelmed, sleep deprived, and uncertain what my baby boy needed, was unsettling. Surely all mothers throughout history didn't begin this way: unprepared and unsupported. Our first six months were a huge challenge, as mother and son struggled to get to know and understand each other. A seed was planted within me, a feeling that life with a newborn could and should be easier—and more fun.

It was seven years before I gave birth again, and I was a different person by then. My son had trained me well, and I was committed to motherhood as my primary function. I was living happily in Hawai'i, and after several years as a single parent, I had a new and loving partner. I was determined to have a homebirth this time, and with the help of a fine midwife-friend, I delivered my beautiful girl after two hours of labor. She went immediately to my breast. My partner was delighted, and served us devotedly as we recuperated from the birth and got to know each other. He provided meals in bed and plenty of fluids, he cared for our older son, and supported us in sleeping, feeding, and following our daughter's rhythms. It was a blissful time; all was well within the small world of family in which we dwelt.

My third birth was less than three years later, and we were back in California. We found a wonderful midwife, and again had a sweet homebirth, receiving another perfect daughter to love. A close friend came for the birth and overnight, taking great care of my older children; but her busy life called her away the next day. I was expecting the same devoted care from my husband that I received after my second birth, but he now had a ten-year old and a two-year old to attend to, and lots of household responsibilities. I remember feeling forgotten and abandoned as the sounds of the household swirled around me. It was sad to realize that the care I expected would not be forthcoming; it was simply more than my man could manage. We had no nearby family members, and our friends were busy with their own responsibilities.

Several years later, my next door neighbor Jill and I were having tea as our children played around us. She was an office manager for our local midwives, and had birthed both her girls at home. After her daughters' births, I had come around to help however I could, making the chicken soup the midwife advised, tidying up, folding laundry, doing errands. Back to work in the midwives' office, Jill mentioned to me that women would occasionally ask if she knew anyone who could help after the baby was born. She told me that she often thought of me as the perfect person for that work. It was a revelation! I was excited by this idea. She shared my phone number and my work began. My youngest was in kindergarten, so I took on one family at a time. As my children grew, my availability expanded. Being a doula has been one of the greatest blessings of my life.

Twenty-five years later, after helping dozens of beautiful newly born babies and parents and after training numerous postpartum doulas, I am filled with experiences and thoughts to share. I have observed a new wave of interest among young women in the field of birth and postpartum care. There is now a need and a desire within our society to increase the joy and create balance and harmony in this period of intense physical and emotional change.

MY GOALS FOR THIS BOOK

I have several goals for this book. First, I want it to serve as a support tool for sisters, mothers, husbands, partners, friends, family, and community members who desire to understand how best to serve the women in their lives who are or will be giving birth. I also write it as a guide to women themselves who want to more fully understand the postpartum experience. I would like to see it used as a text for doula trainings around the world, and as a manual for aspiring postpartum doulas.

Though in some ways a textbook, this guide is a deeply personal and heartfelt sharing of my point of view, gained from years of insight. I have included numerous examples from my own doula practice, spanning twenty-five years, including the words of some of my clients. I speak conversationally at times, and may use "I," "you," "we," or "the doula" when discussing how the caregiver might perform her duties. I have allowed myself inconsistency in this usage; doula work is best performed from the feeling level, and it seems correct to write about it from the same place.

In discussing infants, I have chosen to switch frequently between genders. Sometimes a topic of discussion will remind me of a certain baby and I will gravitate toward use of "he" or "she" according to that child's gender. I have tried to use the gender pronouns fairly equally, without counting, but intending to be inclusive of all infants.

Each chapter is designed to stand alone. Many ideas are repeated, since they are related to more than one topic. For example, the need to help a new breastfeeding mother enjoy pain-free breastfeeding may be discussed not only in "Breastfeeding Support" but also in "Infant Care." This book is intended to be quick reference guide topic by topic, as well as to provide a full picture of the range of postpartum needs.

The *Gentle Art* represents a culmination of the wisdom gleaned from so many wonderful families who opened their homes and hearts to me at this most delicate and sacred time. From each family, I learned more as I strived to give of myself in ways that supported them in finding the magic in their experience.

We are putting out the call to women, and men as well, to care for one another in our times of need. In order to accomplish this on a large scale, we need training, information, and feedback. We require the sharing of wisdom gained through experience. Our wise elders are coming forth to rekindle this light. A shift in attitude and attention is required of the culture, a new honor and respect for birth and life. Birthing mothers can ask for the help they deserve, and educate themselves about what that will be. The intent of this manual is to provide clear, readable, accurate, and useful guidance for friends and family, as well as professional caregivers. What is required is a warm heart and an willingness to serve. The rest is contained within these pages.

SECTION I

THE ART OF CARE

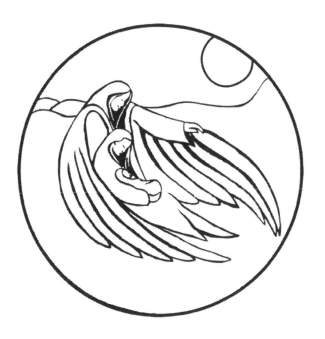

Chapter 1

A SHORT HISTORY OF POSTPARTUM CARE

Birth is a deeply spiritual event, mysterious and miraculous. We honor the child's arrival, in awe of the process that brought it forth. At the same time, birth is profoundly physical, with pain, blood, risk, and no guaranteed outcome. A new mother and her infant are a holy couple, inspiring reverence in all who come near. They are our assurance that human life continues. Yet they are delicate, depleted by the exertions they have undergone, and touched forever by the nature of their birth experience. The mother has been opened to the depths of her being, and the child has been squeezed and pushed and forced into life on Earth. They require careful attention to their physical bodies, as well as sensitivity toward their ever-changing emotions and needs.

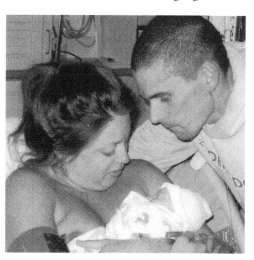

The transition to parenthood is life-changing
—Photo Credit: Salle Webber

Historically, women have cared for one another during these times, guided by intuitive understanding and age-old traditions. A woman and child after birth were cared for by the extended family and neighbors. Food was delivered, older children were cared for, the new mother's needs were tenderly accommodated, and the baby was provided the optimal environment for survival.

As birth has moved into the hospital, it has entered into the realm of the professional, and been removed from normal daily experience. In the Western world, women no longer seem to know innately how to care for one another, assist at birth, or attend to the needs of newborns. As we have chosen to live in nuclear families, no longer are extra adults present in the home to lend a hand in the middle of the night or when mom needs a nap, a shower, a meal, or a willing pair of arms to hold the baby. Many of us have moved away from our families of origin, and more adults have accepted employment outside the home, leaving little time for service to others. Many new mothers have found themselves alone and uninformed, with no designated caregiver or helper. "Postpartum" has almost become synonymous with "depression" in the current vocabulary.

After the initial week or two of devoted attention from partner, family, or friends, a mother may find herself spending long days alone with her child. Isolation and abandonment are feelings common to young mothers, sometimes progressing to what we call postpartum depression. In most cases, this condition can be potentially avoided if the new mom is provided with helpful support, good food, the opportunity to rest a lot, and loving companionship. Physical depletion and sleep deprivation can wreak havoc with the psyche, so as caregivers we strive to provide nourishment and practical care to maximize healing; compassionate emotional support, touched with humor, will calm and assure the new mother that all is well.

THE BIRTH OF A NEW FIELD

"Doula" is a relatively new word for English-speakers, and comes from the Greek language. Dana Raphael first used it in her classic text, *The Tender Gift*, to describe postpartum care providers. It refers to "one who serves," especially in providing care for newborns and their mothers. Another common and wonderful definition is "grandmothering." I love this image because it assumes a caring and involved presence; an attitude that extends beyond a mere job or work situation, and suggests commitment to the long-term well-being of the family. The doula becomes a trusted and integral part of the caregiving team, a confidante and friend, an extension of the family, and one who mothers the new mother.

Doulas can also help during labor. More than 20 years ago, John Kennell, Marshall Klaus, and colleagues designed a study to evaluate the effectiveness of labor support delivered by trained birth doulas (Kennell, Klaus, McGrath, Robertson, & Hinkley, 1991). Women who received this type of support demonstrated faster, less-medicated births, with a significantly lowered c-section rate than those laboring

---

American Heritage Dictionary

doula (doo/la), noun

A woman who assists another woman during labor and provides support to her, the infant, and the family after childbirth. (modern Greek *doula* from Greek dialectical *doula,* servant-woman, slave)

---

without the aid of a doula. Their feelings about the birth experience and their long-term adjustment to mothering were enhanced by the support of trained and compassionate women.

The results of this study were widely publicized, and the word "doula" entered the public domain. Less widely publicized, but still vital, was the work of the postpartum doula, whose service begins after the birth.

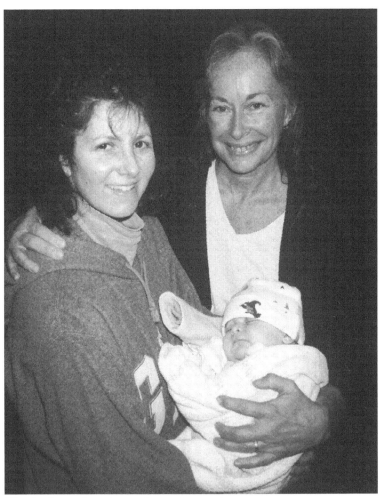

The doula mothers the mother —Photo credit: Gary Young

The postpartum doula steps in after the birth doula's work is finished and the family is on their own, and she is regularly present in the home for several weeks or months. She serves to assist the new parents as they make the tender transition into family life at home. She offers guidance, wisdom, and service, calmly providing physical and emotional nurturing as the mother regains her strength and her infant grows. The postpartum doula cares for the newborn, other children, and the needs of the home. This allows the new mother to rest and heal as she learns to feed and care for her child, developing confidence in her ability to be a successful mother.

It may be difficult to quantify the benefit of a postpartum doula to a new mother. After all, how can you evaluate the effectiveness of breakfast in bed, a clean kitchen, a contented infant, or a shoulder rub? Who knows how long it would take a new mom to heal from a cesarean section birth if she had to do everything herself? How can we evaluate whether the moms who give up on breastfeeding would have persisted with help and encouragement?

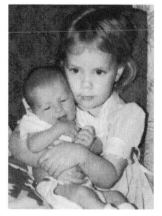

Siblings play a big role in the family's postpartum adjustment —Photo credit: Stacey Dennick

It is utterly fulfilling to witness the organic nature of the newborn family over time. Postpartum doulas are present for the ongoing daily life of the family as it shifts to make room for the new member. It may be difficult to assign a number value to our work, but we can see the difference it makes to each mother we serve; that is rich reward, indeed.

Chapter 2

FIRST-TIME PARENTS

Thank you for being there for me as I made my transition into motherhood. You have provided me with the space and wisdom to love my role as mom, and stay grounded in the most important part of life: family.

—Lou's letter to her doula

When a woman gives birth for the first time, she is forever transformed; the uninitiated young female metamorphoses into full womanhood. She has been entrusted with a baby, and the urgings of her body continue to keep her focused on her new role. Being in constant service to a newborn is unlike any other job she has had, but after nine months of pregnancy, labor and delivery, a woman's body and psyche are attuned to this new life.

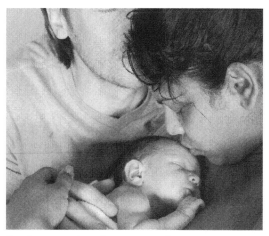

Each generation brings new hope —Photo credit: Maggie Muir.

A father has a somewhat different path. He has a more intellectual idea of the child, not experiencing the intimacy of sharing his body, and it seems that some dads work their way down from head to heart. Not only is he now a father of a helpless infant, but his wife or partner has become someone else. Her emotions are running wild and her focus is entirely on the infant. The new dad may feel overwhelmed with responsibility, both for the newborn and the new mom. He may feel that his own needs are pushed into the background, and his best friend has a new love—the baby.

It is important to take one day at a time, recognizing that each day will be unique. Babies need time to find a rhythm, and at first they are simply responding to physical sensations of hunger, discomfort, and the need to sleep. It is a physiological expectation for human infants to continue the connection with the mother, to be touched and held and spoken to; without this they will be unhappy. The mother, too, needs this contact and intimacy. Babies have shown that they recognize the voices of family members early on, often turning the head toward the sounds they heard from the womb. The family has existed for several months, but they are just now getting acquainted.

Parents need care as they make this huge transition. Planning for a baby and actually having one are very different. The life change that a seven-pound infant can generate is surprising, and it's not something that can be effectively explained to expectant parents. The doula is there to surround them with supportive concern, to help carry the load, empathize, provide practical care as they adapt, and remind them that whatever struggles they're experiencing will pass and that the only constant is change. She will nurture their love for one another.

I've observed the mood swings that can come in the postpartum period. One day the new mom is blissfully in love, the next day she's in tears. She adores her baby, yet feels resentful at times, or overwhelmed with the reality of this huge responsibility. She may feel less than compassionate when the infant screams or poops all over everything. The doula can help by calming and caring for the baby, cleaning up the mess, maintaining her own emotional balance, listening with a compassionate ear, injecting humor where appropriate, and performing small acts of kindness. Remember that new mothers need time during each day to care for themselves. Because we skillfully tend to the infant's needs, the new mother has time to shower and nap, eat a meal, make a phone call, or sit outside in the sun. Her life has changed drastically, and some days she may find no opportunity to brush her teeth or hair, take her vitamins, eat an actual meal, or talk to her partner. This is especially true for first-time mothers, who have not developed habits of motherhood and are struggling with this demanding new role. An understanding ear can help; compassion is the healer.

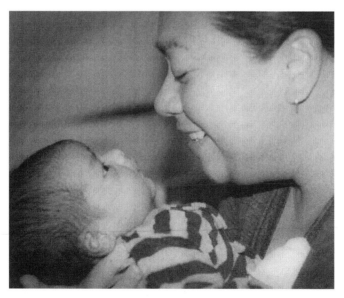

New motherhood inspires feelings of deep love and connection
—Photo credit: Jeannine Marshall

We can support her transition in practical ways: by inviting her to nap, offering to change a diaper or bring up a burp, providing clean and folded laundry. Many moms enjoy closing the door to the bedroom and being completely alone for a while. Others need to talk it out, to express the confusion in words. After a few weeks of healing, a couple of hours out with a friend or mate can rejuvenate a weary mommy. This will be easy to accomplish if the new mom has complete trust in her doula's ability to lovingly care for her infant.

The new parents need time together to reconnect and nurture each other. The doula can observe moments of opportunity to quietly carry the infant into another room, allowing his parents some private time. Several mothers have complained to me that they miss the physical contact with their partners as they sleep, since the baby is now sleeping between them. It is easy for these couples to get disconnected in slow and subtle ways. I like to remind moms to encourage the partner's participation by handing the baby to him to hold, including him as a helper in nursing rituals, and discussing her observations of their baby with him. They are traveling this path together, and though it may be rocky and windy, it is well to travel as a team, in cooperation and shared commitment. The foundation for this unified experience is laid in these early months.

I sometimes suggest the parents take a nap together when I'm available for infant care, or go for a short walk or out to lunch. This is a tender, wonderful, and difficult time for these individuals. No experience can really prepare a person for parenthood, and it comes on full force. Helping them ease into these new roles is an act of kindness. We can provide the parents with short breaks, or respite from the non-stop responsibility of newborn care—a chance to catch their breath, to regroup before continuing on.

The birth of a baby generates absolute responsibility for another human being, and this is not an easy role to accept: making the needs of another person more important than one's own needs represents a huge life change. I used to tell my first-born, "You taught me everything I know about being a mom." The lessons were not always easy. I take these memories with me into the homes of first-time parents, where I feel compassion and kindness toward their inner struggles. I refrain from judging and strive to model competent, effective baby care—ways of soothing and handling the infant that parents can copy successfully. I have often been told, "I was doing the Salle-bounce in the middle of the night."

You modeled a very nurturing and gentle way to be with a baby, something that I didn't have a clue about at that point.
—Sheila's letter to her doula

The ideal doula for first-time parents is one who is expert in infant care. She can demonstrate holding and comforting techniques, handling the child confidently and comfortably, always with head support and a firm but tender hand. This will provide a visual guide to the new parents. Maintaining a soft voice and a body free of excess tension will allow the baby to relax. Keeping the infant calm during diapering and dressing is a useful skill they can learn with the doula's support. Essentially, what we want to impart to our new parents is a growing sense of empowerment, a recognition that the answers to the questions their children bring are already inside of them; that they are capable of parenting; that they can trust themselves to do OK. And when it feels difficult, that too is OK. As the parents develop an understanding of the newborn's "language," they are able to respond more confidently, quickly relieving their infant's crying. This provides a growing sense of mastery over this new reality. Assisting parents to gain these infant-care skills is a vital part of our service.

Helping new parents establish boundaries may be necessary, especially if their circle of friends is mostly childless. Some people don't understand the focus required by family life, and complain of hearing too much about diapers, feedings, and middle-of-the-night episodes. They want their old friend back; alas, that old friend no longer exists. I've been asked to screen phone calls, telling the caller the mom is sleeping, or explaining why she can't go to the beach or to a party. I've met friends at the door, waylaying their attempt to barge into a quiet breastfeeding session or disturb a resting mother. I'm a professional; I can do that.

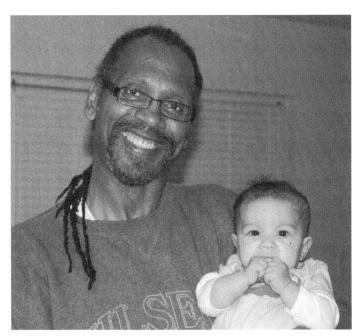

The extended family and community welcomes its newest member and offers practical support to the new parents —Photo credit: Jason Peters-Smith

Grandparents and other family members can sometimes cause distress to new parents, especially if they are highly opinionated, disrespectful of the young parents' choices, or needy instead of helpful when visiting. There are many beliefs and lifestyles doulas will come into contact with, and we respect them all. However, our loyalty is to the family we are serving, and we politely defend their right to make their own decisions. In many cases, I have been asked to provide care for the first month or more, until the new parents feel secure and comfortable in their role. Then they are willing to invite the grandparents, after they have become the experienced and competent mother and father of this grandchild.

The advantage of the doula is that she has no agenda other than service, no need to push her opinions, and no complex history with either parent that can cloud the moment. It is important for each family to find its own way, its own rhythm and style, without judgment or pressure, but with support and encouragement. Whether or not the extended family provides this nurturing environment, the help of a skilled doula is invaluable.

Chapter 3

CARING FOR NEWBORN FAMILIES

Thank you so much for your incredible care. You made the amazing richness so much smoother. I will forever be grateful for your kind, healing ways.

—Catherine, first-time mom

You made a difference in the joy and peace of our home. You will forever be part of our happy memories surrounding the birth of our daughter.

—Simone, to her doula

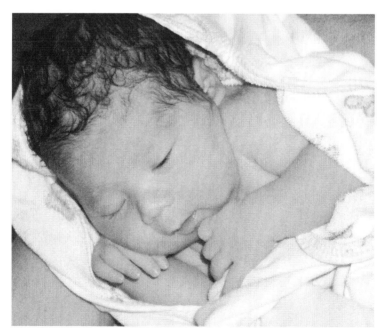

The newborn opening to his world —Photo credit: Blaine Michioka

The newborn is a multifaceted being. Pure as a new day, his flesh never before exposed to air, his tiny features appearing both innocent and wise, he exists somewhere between the Earth and the heavens. His family has made the leap of faith to open itself to receive this new life. They love him without even knowing him. This in itself is a miracle! Birth is surely a holy experience, stirring us to states of awe and reverence.

Yet, this is a profoundly physical event. The intensity and complexity of factors insist that we approach birth with skill and knowledge. The mother's body is hugely challenged, and physical emergencies can arise. The child is going through a hard journey where risks exist, and everything must work together for a successful outcome. The physical aspect of birth is necessarily prioritized.

This dichotomy continues in the days following the birth. We are filled with the miraculous as we gaze upon the tiny infant, but then, sticky, black meconium seeps out onto the blanket, and the new mother bleeds onto the sheets. The child cries. Hunger? Discomfort? Need to be held? This routine is repeated day and night. Sleep deprivation sets in.

Mom's perineum may be tender. Her nipples may be sensitive to the child's suck, and baby may struggle and fuss as she strives to learn to nurse. Everyone is hungry or thirsty. Dirty laundry piles up. Chores go undone. Ordinary daily life demands our ongoing attention.

The stage is set for the entrance of the doula, whether a professional or the helpful friend or family member. Our role is service. The doula sees to it that everyone is fed, the bed is clean, and soiled items disappear from sight and reappear later, clean and dry. We assist the mother and newborn as they figure out breastfeeding and find their way back to sleep. We may prepare a sitz bath with healing herbs for a sore perineum, or provide the parents with an opportunity to nap or reconnect with each other.

The baby needs to be observed, as well, for signs of thriving: poopy diapers, successful feedings, and moments of alertness that gradually get longer. The doula recognizes jaundice, may observe thrush, and can comment on rashes. We always recommend checking with the medical practitioner for anything unusual, and are clear that we're not nurses, but experienced mothers. Midwives have told me that the first five days are critical, and I keep this awareness, as I make sure

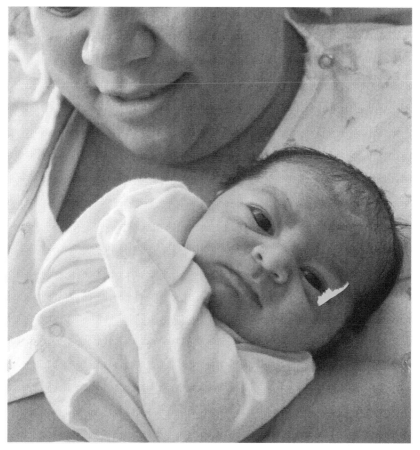

Periods of alertness characterize the healthy newborn —Photo credit: Jeannine Marshall

the newborn is warm enough, waking every few hours to eat, and "checked on" frequently.

In fact, the baby at this time is still transitioning between worlds. He needs human touch, voices, and the stimulation of skin-to-skin contact to remind him of his new place in life. We must draw him into worldly existence with our attention, love, and enthusiasm for his presence among us.

There have been times when parents have told me of a late-night crying episode that they were sure had no physical cause. We do not know what emotional and intellectual experiences the infant may have, what awareness he has of past and future, what fears he may be holding. We must strive to be truly sensitive to this state. The infant is not an empty body, waiting to be filled by the environment we put it in. Rather, the infant is a spiritual being having an earthly experience: here to manifest particular qualities, tendencies, and abilities, and to move on in his personal evolution. You and I, the caregivers, are willing servants of this process, smoothing the path and easing any suffering we can. It is a wonderful role to play, drawing forth our most compassionate hearts, as we gaze on the innocent and helpless infant.

The condition known as SIDS, Sudden Infant Death Syndrome, often occurs when babies are separated from their parents and sleeping in their own room. The first six months of life are the most vulnerable. It is vital that the child be near its caretakers, can hear voices or breathing, and be looked at and listened to regularly. We know that some babies cease breathing and pass on for no apparent reason. Perhaps the isolation is more than they can bear. Some experts theorize that the breathing mechanism of the infant needs to be re-stimulated periodically by the sound, touch, or smell of another human being. If the child is alone, the breath may simply cease.

It is not my intention to discuss the causes of SIDS, but to point out the importance of mothers staying very connected with their babies. It's a mutual need of both infant and mother. The hormones of love and attachment are flowing. This is the time to bond deeply and fully, physically, and spiritually. It is a gift that will last a lifetime.

More women are recognizing the value of mother's milk and committing themselves to breastfeeding their infants. Developing a

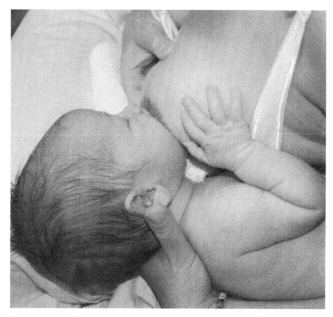

As every nursing couple is unique, finding a comfortable breastfeeding position is essential —Photo credit: Maggie Muir

successful nursing relationship is vital. Learning the art of breastfeeding can hold challenges for both mother and baby; calm support and encouragement at this stage can make the difference between peaceful and stressful feeding. There are certain basics that all doulas need to understand (outlined in "Breastfeeding Support" chapter), and we can make a huge difference in the family's experience by sharing our patience and knowledge.

We can also make the feeding session easier by offering to hold the baby while mother puts away the first breast and readies the second, or changing a diaper during a break. We can ensure mom has water nearby when she sits down to nurse, as well as pillows if she needs them, and we can lend assistance in getting comfortable. When a mother is well-fed, watered, and rested, she feels better able to breastfeed successfully. This is absolutely primary; it is about physical survival. Sure, supermarket infant formula is available, and the baby can survive without breast milk. But on a profound level it feeds a woman's soul to nurture her child with her body, naturally. Many women experience deep disappointment if they do not nurse their babies, regardless of the reason. We know that breast milk provides exactly what's required at each stage of the baby's life; the initial colostrum, packed with antibodies, being the first golden layer of protection for life on Earth.

If the child is not breastfeeding, she will receive formula, or perhaps donor-breast milk, from a bottle or other feeding device. Caregivers can assist with bottle-feedings, taking care to feed patiently and unhurriedly.

Settling into a comfortable feeding routine is essential to having a happy baby, and a relaxed mommy. Establishing the ability to feed the newborn with relative ease is a high priority of the initial week or two after birth.

The new mother's body has gone through a tremendous experience for the sake of this child. She has sacrificed personal comfort and made the needs of another her highest priority, and she must continue to do so. She must feed the child 8 to 12 times a day, round the clock, with never a day off. She must surrender her own needs and desires as she cares for the infant, only sleeping or eating between feedings, diaper changes, rocking, and soothing. Anything we can do to smooth her path, lighten her load, or touch her spirit, is beneficial. She is wide-open, highly sensitive, and delicate. She is also fiercely protective and instinctive. She merits our respect and honor. Allow her to be cared for like a queen for a while. She deserves it. The doula can set the tone, by letting family members know what they can do to support mom, and enlisting them into her care.

As the old saying goes, "If Mama ain't happy, ain't nobody happy!" Many of us can vouch for that, especially at this time of hormonal upheaval and extreme physical demand.

My bottom-line day-to-day philosophy of the work of a doula is to meet the needs of the mother, whether it be for food or drink; to have her kitchen cleaned or her children fed; to be listened to as she shares her birth story, her dissatisfactions, or her bliss. Perhaps it's the laundry needing to be folded and put away, her baby held so she can nap, or some time to be alone. Whatever she needs, I know it will support her healing and recuperation if I can tune in and serve her. If mom's needs are met, she's better able to give of herself to her baby, her partner, and family. This is my ultimate goal: to support harmony, health, and satisfaction in the postpartum circle.

Chapter 4

THE NEEDS OF THE POSTPARTUM MOTHER

POSTPARTUM CARE IN TRADITIONAL CULTURES

In traditional and tribal cultures, mother and child are cared for, sheltered and protected for up to 40 days after birth. Women of the community attend to their personal needs, and care for the home and family. Generally the mother and infant don't leave the home during that time. It is well understood that this period is delicate, baby's life is tenuous, and the mother needs to rebuild her strength to feed and care for her child in the years ahead.

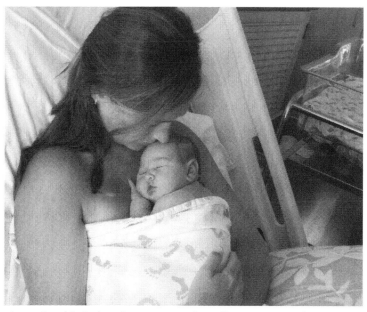

A comfortable bed and a content infant allow a new mother to enjoy and reflect on her new reality —Photo credit: Maggie Muir

To the tribe, each life is valuable, and they work together to provide the best possible outcome, knowing that life can slip away quickly. With our modern medical facilities, we often fail to recall what a tremendous miracle it is to undergo pregnancy and childbirth, and to raise a child. We expect successful outcomes, yet the possibilities of complications are vast, as our foremothers knew all too well. It is prudent to treat the postpartum weeks in a tender and careful way, as an investment in the long-term health and well-being of mother and child.

POSTPARTUM CARE IN MODERN SETTINGS

Though the traditions of mother-care vary throughout the world, a woman who has just given birth requires certain basic necessities: the need for a safe and clean nest for herself and her baby; fluids to replace those lost in childbirth; nourishing food to replenish her body; and plenty of rest to accommodate the baby's need for around-the-clock feeding. If we keep these few things in mind, we will be serving the essential needs shared by all mothers.

In the first few days postpartum, up to two weeks in some cases, mother and baby will mostly be snuggled in bed together. The mother should be encouraged to get up only when she feels like it, and provided with food and drink. One wonderful female doctor recommends, especially after surgical birth, two weeks in the bed, two weeks on the bed, and two weeks near the bed. Frequently, I ask if mom would like clean sheets on her bed. This may be necessary on a daily basis. This is a time of bodily fluids: breast milk dripping, lochia[1] flowing, baby pee and poop leaking out of diapers.

[1]Lochia: the discharge from the uterus following childbirth, which may continue for several weeks.

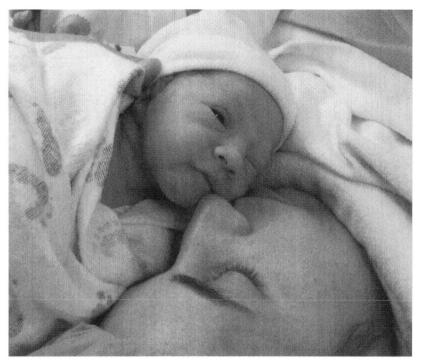

Two weeks in the bed, two weeks on the bed, two weeks near the bed…after a surgical birth —Photo credit: Natasha Joyet

To reduce clutter and provide a calm ambiance, doulas tidy up around the room, pick up dirty clothes and dishes, throw away obvious trash, and straighten piles of books and magazines. Try to create an environment that is restful to eye and soul, that will allow the new mom to dwell on the beauty of her child without material distraction. It is also helpful to see that the things she needs, such as her water, a snack, phone, magazine or book, are in easy reach. These simple acts will make a big difference.

Sharon is a rock in her community, one who others come to for advice and support. When she delivered her third child, it was a difficult birth. She lost a significant amount of blood, and was physically and emotionally exhausted. As her doula, I found her in bed looking quite disheveled and uncomfortable, her older children appearing lost without the attention of the capable and devoted mother they were used to. I herded the kids into the kitchen, fixed them breakfast, and went back to Sharon. She was instantly relieved to have a bit of the pressure taken off, and said she wanted nothing more than to sleep. I bundled her newborn girl onto my chest, threw a load of laundry into the washer, and moved the energetic youngsters into the other end of the house. I engaged the older children in drawing, then in the game of sorting laundry. They played outside for a while as their mom slept deeply. About the time the baby began to stir, Sharon awoke, feeling that tingling in her breasts. After a session of nursing, I brought her a tray of warm and nourishing food. I held the infant while she ate and checked in with her other children. Friends came by to invite the older ones to the park to play. Once the house was quiet, Sharon took a leisurely shower, during which time I changed her sheets and tidied up her bedroom. She returned from her shower and uttered a cry of joy to see her bed so welcoming! Little things mean a lot at times like this. She crawled right in.

It took two weeks for Sharon to begin feeling well, and she spent her time close to her bed. I worked to ease her burden by tending the other children's needs, keeping the laundry moving, and holding her baby. I encouraged her to take care of herself, to enjoy long showers and good food and drink, and to allow members of her community to assist her family by bringing meals, entertaining the children, helping with shopping, and stopping by for an hour to do whatever needed to be done. Many women are so used to taking care of everyone else, they hardly remember

how to honor their own needs. It was a reminder for Sharon
that we all need each other, and she surrendered gracefully to the
demands of her own body.

SIMPLE NECESSITIES

Fluids

Abundant fluids are vital to the postpartum body. Not only has the birthing woman lost blood and fluids during the delivery, she is the sole producer of food for her newborn. This puts a constant demand on her body. Offer water or herbal tea or, if she prefers, diluted juice, continuously. When she sits down to nurse, be sure she has a drink within easy reach once she gets settled.

Remind her frequently to drink. Herbal teas, such as Mothers' Milk Blend, will encourage lactation. In cases of low iron levels, yellow dock root can strengthen the blood. This is especially beneficial after cesarean birth. Fennel tea consumed by the mother can help to reduce gas in baby's tummy. Chamomile or lemon balm can be soothing to the stomach, and are delicious. In some cases, the mother will appreciate her doula brewing up a large pot of tea to last the day. Some women prefer juice, which should be diluted by half. Juice is concentrated, has high sugar content, and can produce heartburn or gas. Even all-natural juices can be over-stimulating, so diluting is a great solution. Many women prefer drinking plain pure water. It should be taken abundantly, at least a full glass for each feeding, and drinking whenever thirsty throughout the day.

As headaches can be a result of dehydration, I first consider her fluid intake when a new mom complains of this ailment. It is not uncommon for a mother to forget to drink as much water as her body requires. Frequent reminders to drink are an appropriate part of postpartum care, and I make it my business to place a fresh glass of water within reach of a nursing mother.

Feeding Mom

Mothers don't typically have big appetites for a few days after giving birth, but that generally changes when their milk comes in and the caloric demands on their bodies go up dramatically. It is generally agreed that a breastfeeding woman needs at least five hundred extra calories daily (Eiger & Olds, 1999; Huggins, 2005). Wholesome, nutritious, simple foods are required. Protein is essential. "Empty calories" in excess are discouraged.

A woman may become ravenously hungry as the demands of milk production escalate. She should be offered nutritious snacks throughout the day, every two to three hours. It is often difficult to eat an actual meal when caring for an infant, so frequent snacking can be an effective substitute. Encourage the family to stock up on easy-to-eat finger foods, such as cut-up melons or carrots, granola bars, cheese sticks, cooked meats, nuts, dried fruits, whole-grain crackers, apples, bananas, and berries. Warming leftovers is a great way to get a quick and tasty mini-meal. A new mother needs to be able to feed herself with one hand, standing up!

If a new mom is not breastfeeding, she still requires strengthening meals. She has also lost fluids during birth, and needs plenty of liquids. Her caloric intake, however, does not require the increase necessary for milk production, and some formula-feeding moms find it harder to lose the weight gained in pregnancy. It is helpful to support her in eating well and exercising gently to begin her return to a fit body.

Families in America, certainly in my community of Santa Cruz, California, have a wide variety of eating styles and preferences, including numerous ethnic variations. I honor each family's choices and work within their comfort zone. It is not in my job description to tell people what I think they should eat. It is, however, my job to offer a salad or cut-up fresh fruit, or to make a sandwich, and would you like lettuce on that? People who eat a lot of processed foods are often happy to eat freshly prepared food if someone else makes it. This is a good time to support excellent nutrition, but never in a preachy way. I find that many people welcome a willing cook into the kitchen, and it is most helpful to offer to prepare meals and snacks at this important and demanding time. Nourishing the mother's body is essential to her healing, her long-term recovery and adjustment, her psychological state, and in support of breastfeeding.

The ideal foods for a nursing mother are fresh, organically grown if possible, minimally processed, and easily digestible. If a food causes gastric distress to the mother it may also upset the infant, and should be avoided. A balance of vegetables, proteins, complex carbohydrates, and fruits is ideal. If an infant experiences regular severe distress, the mother may try eliminating dairy products and wheat from her diet. We have historically recommended minimizing certain gas-producing foods, but science has shown that while a mother's diet can influence her baby, it is not nearly as much as we once thought; breast milk is made from what is in the bloodstream, not in the mother's digestive tract. Newborns may be unsettled in the early weeks, and this may show up as fussiness after feeding. In any case, simple, whole, somewhat bland foods are best for the early weeks. Good nutritional balance is essential. Caffeine and alcohol should be avoided or minimized. At the same time, mothers don't need to feel deprived of all their favorite treats. An occasional chocolate cookie, tiny glass of wine, or half cup of coffee may help her state of mind.

Personal Care

> *You always soothed me … I felt like I was in the best hands,*
> *but you didn't dote on me and make me feel like an invalid. And*
> *I could take a shower!*
>
> —Jesse, mother of twins

A new mother is grateful for an opportunity to bathe, brush and floss her teeth, wash and dry her hair. This is only possible if a competent and trusted person is available to care for her newborn. Then she can indulge herself in a long and delicious shower, attending to the cares of her body. She needs time to gaze in the mirror, to examine the changes in her body since birth, to reconnect with herself.

Sitz baths are also helpful, particularly where there has been perineal tearing or stitching, or hemorrhoids. A convenient plastic tub which fits on the toilet seat is available at drug stores, and provided to patients at some hospitals. Warm water is soothing, but herbal combinations that nourish and heal the perineal tissue are even better, and can be found in health food stores. The doula can prepare the herbs and have them hot when mom is ready, adding cold water to perfect the temperature for this soothing, relaxing experience.

I often remind women who have just given birth that their abdominal organs have been pushed around to accommodate the growing womb. Now that the baby is out, the organs can return to their proper position. This is best facilitated by spending time lying on the back, allowing the organs to settle deep in the inner cavity, as the muscles contract to hold them in place. If a woman is constantly upright, those organs tend to fall forward, and find a new place due to the pull of gravity. This results in the protruding belly common to mothers. Some women recognize this as a good reason to rest, allowing gravity to assist their full healing and return to a non-pregnant body.

Sleep

A general rule of thumb says that a woman should strive to get as much sleep each 24 hours as she was used to getting at night in her pre-pregnant life. In other words, naps are essential. Sleep will definitely be disturbed every few hours all night, every night, for a good while. This is not a problem that needs to be solved. It is the appropriate feeding schedule for a newborn, and we must adapt to it. The infant's stomach is roughly the size of her fist, so she can receive only a small amount per feeding. Breast milk is wonderfully digestible, and needs to be replenished frequently. Moms need to be encouraged to go with the flow, not to strive to create a child who sleeps through the night early, but to accept the reality of her baby's needs and shift her own schedule for awhile. We Americans try hard to be efficient and structured, but babies know no nationality and can only be who they are. We encourage moms to lie down with their baby to sleep during the day, go to bed early at night, and certainly to take the opportunity to sleep when the doula is present to care for baby and home.

Particularly if there are siblings needing care, napping can be a challenge. Again, here the doula can really help. I've often bundled the just-fed, sleepy baby onto my chest and gathered up siblings for a good long walk while mamma basks in the luxury of a quiet house. As the postpartum weeks pass, we may attend a mother less often, perhaps twice a week. She will look forward to the visit, knowing that even if she feels exhausted, once her doula arrives, she can count on a period of complete relaxation. It can help her get through the hard

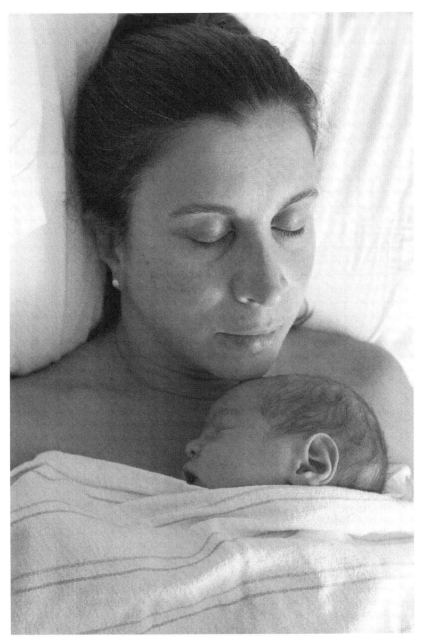

Quiet naps with baby help a new mom to get the rest she needs while staying connected to her newborn —Photo credit: Alan Peevers

hours, knowing help is on the way. Truly, a doula or a trusted and competent friend can be a beacon of light and hope for a tired, busy postpartum woman.

FEEDING CHOICES

The decision of whether or not to breastfeed has many ramifications, not just for the health of the infant. Nursing a newborn supports the healing of the postnatal woman's body by helping to contract extended abdominal muscles, curtailing bleeding, contracting the uterus, and supporting weight loss and return to a non-pregnant body.

It is important to mention that formula-fed babies often sleep for longer periods of time than breastfed babies. This is because formula is a heavier, slower-to-digest food, giving the child a longer period of feeling full. Breast milk composition varies from hour to hour. Mom and baby are intimately connected, as they were in the womb. This is the way it's supposed to be. On-demand feedings are appropriate, as we can't really say how much the baby received last feeding. With formula, I've often observed that the baby isn't hungry again for three to four hours, almost like clockwork. With proper mixing, formula is exactly the same every time, and provides a rather predictable feeding schedule.

Some couples decide to give dad one of the night feedings, allowing mom a longer stretch of sleep. In some cases the decision is made in a breastfeeding situation to supplement with formula once or twice a day to give mom a break and to share the feeding ritual with other relatives. With the current popularity of breast pumps, some women keep a small supply of breast milk for this purpose.

These are personal decisions for parents to make. I may feel very strongly about the superiority of breast milk over formula, and there is lots of evidence to support this. However, the emotional and psychological factors involved in parenting are complex and profound, and it is not the doula's place to challenge the couple's beliefs, but only to support the fulfillment of their needs. We accept that this child came to these parents, needing what they have to offer. We desire the highest and best for each baby and family, but we don't decide what that actually is. We are there to serve and uplift, to bring comfort and harmony, however that may manifest.

In that spirit, if we are asked to feed the baby a bottle while mom sleeps, goes to the dentist, takes a walk with husband or friend, or works at her computer, we gladly do just that, with love in our hearts. The peace of mind of the mother is more important to the child, perhaps, than the precise diet she receives. I can't emphasize enough the importance of support, not judgments, and of allowing the family to find its own way. As the parents become empowered, they will make clearer choices for their family, knowing what is appropriate for them. We never want to suggest that they are not doing it the way we think is right. On the contrary, our goal is to help them feel empowered to successfully perform this work of parenting. It is the highest service we can offer.

MOTHERS' NEEDS

Emotional Needs

A woman's estrogen and progesterone levels, so high for many months, drop dramatically after the birth. The production of stress hormones increases, as the mother's weary body strives to keep up with the demands of the newborn and the expectations of those around her. This frequently peaks around the third to fifth days postpartum, which are well-known for emotional sensitivity. I always prepare myself for the possibility of being greeted with tears and frustration on these days, when for some women their balance is temporarily lost.

Beyond this, doulas see emotional upheavals related to the common expectations of our culture. This birth represents a huge change in a woman's life. More will be demanded of her than ever before—she is in an emotional whirlpool. Her child inspires feelings she's never known were possible, deep love and tenderness, as well as overwhelm and self-doubt. She finds herself playing a role for which she may have had no rehearsal; yet everyone seems to think she should play the part effortlessly!

While friends and family are thrilled about the new baby, they are very busy in their own lives. The new mom may find herself spending

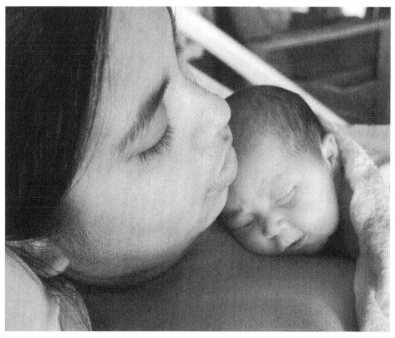

Birth brings momentous responsibility and profound change —Photo credit: Maggie Muir

hours at a time alone at home with her newborn. She may be coming from a fast-paced job with lots of stimulation, or a full social life, and now spends hours walking the floor hoping to put the baby to sleep, often in her pajamas all day, forgetting when she last brushed her teeth. It is vital to retain perspective at this time, to know this is temporary and precious. Postpartum depression threatens as a mom may begin to feel her own needs unmet. She requires compassion and humor, and small breaks from her responsibilities. The need for a helpful companion who shares concern for the family is a role the doula fills naturally. She is capable, confident, friendly and willing to engage fully in the life of the household. She understands the mother's fragile state, and serves to make her feel comfortable and appreciated, acknowledging the great importance of the mother's role.

> *Kim had help from her husband and her mother, but she commented that emotional ties and old behavior patterns can take their toll. With a professional doula, there were no strings attached—she didn't have to treat her like a guest, care for her needs or invest emotional energy into what she found to be a very non-demanding relationship. Aside from the physical help, Kim felt that she benefited from her doula's attitude, which she described as "proud to do women's work, serene in her chosen path."*
>
> —From *Who Needs a Doula* by Laurie Dodge

Calm and experienced support can be extremely reassuring. A short break from the responsibility of the baby can do wonders for a mother's perspective. In some cases, just the simple presence of a friendly adult woman is enough to keep a new mom going in what can

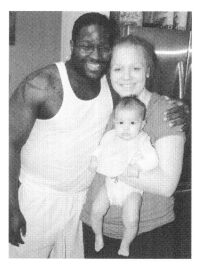

The participation of her partner and their warm emotional bond, support a new mother's well-being
—Photo credit: James Cox

seem at times like a roller coaster of endless demands and responsibilities in an isolated world.

The Need to Understand: Fussy Baby/Frustrated Parents

Feelings of inadequacy often come up as new parents struggle to learn their baby's signals. Any fussiness on the baby's part causes them to feel they're doing something wrong, or the baby doesn't like them. Mothers are especially prone to these concerns, as they are often associated with feeding. As discussed in the chapter "Breastfeeding Support," several new moms I've worked with were responding to squirming and fussing at the breast with the conviction that they didn't have enough milk, sure that the baby was hungry and frustrated. I suggested that they consider the possibility that their babies were reacting to their own body's sensations, such as gas bubbles moving through, or the need to poop. I encouraged them to pick their babies up and attempt to soothe them by rubbing or gently patting their backs. Generally, a burp would come soon, or a bowel movement, and the feeding could continue.

Moms need to learn not to take it personally when the baby is unhappy. I have often explained that the child is adapting to life in this body, with immature organs and systems, and she feels many sensations that may be uncomfortable. She has no choice but to respond to these discomforts with fussing, crying, or squirming. She has very little control over her body and needs our help to burp, fart, get comfortable, go to sleep, and stay warm.

The challenge is to learn to recognize what the baby is expressing. Most mothers are fast learners, as they are involved all day every day with the baby. The doula can share her baby wisdom, to help the parents understand their child's needs, and to offer tools for dealing with difficult moments. We acknowledge the parents for their newfound awareness about their infant, and point out the many things they have learned, how far they have come. We want to build their confidence in themselves as parents, recognizing that they are the ones who know their child the best, and that they can call upon their intuitive understanding regarding what's right for their beloved babies. Learning to trust oneself as a parent is a giant step.

The Need to Have Her Home and Family Cared For

As discussed more fully in later chapters, in order to truly relax, a postpartum woman needs to know that her home is being well cared for. If she has older children, she will be distracted from her restful state if their needs are not being met. If her home is tidy and her children are happy, she can relax and focus on the new life in her arms. By being friendly and open, not forcing ourselves on small children who don't know us well, but offering food, help, or companionship, we can win their trust. We may offer to read a story, take a walk, or invite the child to help with folding laundry or washing dishes. Perhaps he'd like to draw pictures together or do a simple art project. Asking to see his room may generate play, or sharing. Becoming a trusted friend to her child is a way to provide great relief to a postpartum mother. Non-professional helpers may already have a close relationship to the child, and can provide a huge service by devoting time and attention to his needs.

THE TRAUMA OF MEDICAL EMERGENCY

If a newborn requires emergency medical intervention, we can be sure that his mother is in emotional distress, as well. She has undergone labor and delivery, or surgery to birth the baby, and is herself in need of rest and attention. Her hormones are beginning their descent, her breasts are throbbing with the urge to suckle her child, and she has given her infant into the care of strangers she must trust with his well-being. The worry is enormous, and there may be feelings of guilt and responsibility for whatever problems are occurring.

If the newborn is hospitalized for days or weeks, the parents are trekking between hospital and home daily. The mother may be pumping her breasts to maintain her milk supply and to provide nourishment that her child receives through a tube, syringe, or bottle. This is physically and emotionally taxing. There is great frustration in watching one's infant lie in isolation, with IV hookups, tubes and catheters, being unable to hold or comfort the child. Sometimes it feels impossible to recognize the tiny being as one's own, generating internal confusion. It is a tense and fearful time, and can tax the relationship between the parents, as they each wrestle with their emotions. Ideally, this event will strengthen the bond between the mother and father of the struggling infant, as they cling to one another for comfort, but this is not always the case. There may be subtle elements of guilt or blame that can enormously complicate the process.

As the doula in such circumstances, we are generally not present until the infant is finally brought home. This may be several weeks into his life. There is joy in the release from the hospital, signifying the physical stability of the baby, but there may be apprehension about the new level of responsibility for this fragile little one. The parents are suddenly put into the role of full-time caregivers, with no more assistance from nurses and hospital personnel. They must work cooperatively to meet their infant's needs. The doula should see the parents as delicate, too, and in need of nurturing, rest, and understanding.

Baby Dylan was born early and hospitalized in the Newborn Intensive Care Unit. When he was finally released to his parents' care, his mother, Shannon, expressed that she and Scott felt as if they had adopted Dylan; the doctor and nurses had been in charge of him for almost three months before he came home, he seemed to belong to them.

This transition can be daunting, as parents find themselves responsible for every aspect of baby's care. It is up to them now to decipher the infant's needs, to respond to his signals. They may call on their doula for clarity, and modeling warm and compassionate baby-handling is appropriate. Show them how to gently accommodate him, speaking softly, with lots of touch and gentle massage. His body may be tense from receiving frequent injections or IV needles, blood draws, tubes in his nose or throat. He may require re-patterning, to be able to relax his body. We accomplish this with hours of patiently holding the baby, whispering soothing sounds, rocking or swaying, encouraging him to release the tension in his little body. Healing is always possible.

For the parents, lots of encouragement and affirmation of their accomplishments is helpful. Point out the little successes you see each day, the signs of continuing growth and development. Be attentive to the details. Recognize that the parents, too, are delicate and in need of TLC. Feed them, tidy up around them, do their laundry, encourage them to rest. Model for them how to soothe and care tenderly for their infant. Regardless of the age of the newborn, the postpartum period really gets going when the little family goes home and begins to create their own structure. Encourage bonding, napping together, lengthy suckling, cuddling, snuggling in bed as a family, luxuriating in the softness and warmth of skin-to-skin contact. Don't skip over the tender days just because of medical interruption; begin at the beginning, with special care for mother and child, honoring their journey and welcoming the newborn into his world.

JEANE'S STORY

I found myself pregnant at 44! One of the best miracles in my life was having my son at home in a tub of water, surrounded by my best girlfriends. I do not think I could have had such a pleasant journey if it hadn't been for their support. One of my most special sisters, Salle, is a doula. I am an old fashioned kind of a thinker when it comes to having babies. I have always thought it was best to have them at home with all the women around for help, with a strong midwife. I always believed it was best to have help for a couple of months after the baby is born to help the family integrate, and to help with overcoming postpartum blues, which I experienced with my second child. In my theory, postpartum blues come from not sleeping and not having help with the baby and the rest of your responsibilities as your body is adjusting.

This is where Salle came into her service. Salle was at my son's birth. She was right there with me the whole way. She slept on the couch and was right there the first time my infant son nursed. She was so helpful, watching with her expert eye, making sure my son was latched on just right. Salle took my mind off of all the other responsibilities I had going on. With two other children in school and a busy husband, who was going to do laundry or make sure there was a snack ready for the kids coming home from school, keep up with grocery shopping and light house work? This is where a new momma needs support.

Salle is so perfect in this role as doula. Her work is soft and sweet. While I was nursing my son, she would prepare a light lunch for me and let me spend time with my newborn. Afterward Salle would see to it that I had a bath, clean pajamas on, and she tucked me tenderly into bed. Meanwhile the laundry would be going and somehow the kids were all home from school. The household was running very smoothly. I could sleep so well during this time because Salle would hold my baby the whole time I was napping, I did not ever have any worry on my mind; I was totally able to relax. After a good three hours or so Salle would bring my cuddly baby to me, ready to nurse. Salle took the time to see that we were both comfortable and off she would go to fix me a bite to eat. Salle always made sure I was drinking enough water and taking all of the supplements my midwife ordered for me. I really loved having this kind of help. Ease of mind is important during the first few months, to help create a new pattern naturally. Having a new baby can be so stressful to the entire family, but with effective support, this does not have to be so.

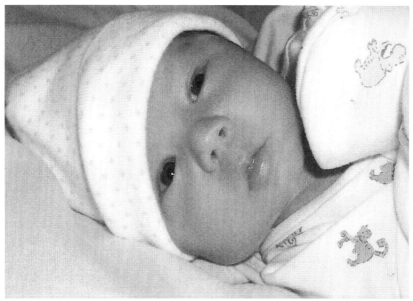

Jeane's son at five days old —Photo credit: Blaine Michioka

Chapter 5

MOTHER-MODELING

Thank you for your flexibility and willingness to be with what was going on in our household … you modeled skills for me that I still employ …

— Barbara, mother of two

I feel honored to witness the process new parents go through as they are transformed by the birth and postpartum experiences. It is as if the ego dies and is reborn into parenthood. So many discoveries are made, large and small, about who we really are and what is truly important in this life.

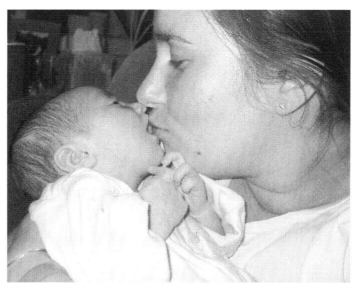

The intimacy that began in the womb continues as a love affair of mother and child —Photo credit: Darrin MacLeod

A parent's awareness is alchemized through witnessing the miracle of their own child emerging from the womb. While observing the infant, caring for her, becoming intimate with this immaculate new person, the parent grows immensely in the ability to express unconditional love. This is certainly one of the treasured opportunities of earthly life: we get to feel our hearts opened and willingly give ourselves to the service of another human being, to set aside our own needs in favor of the beloved child. Even marriage does not bring full selflessness in this way. The helplessness, purity, and innocence of the newborn brings us to this place of total love, a place we may never have known existed within us.

At the same time, the dependent infant's demands can be confusing and overwhelming, coming at all hours of night and day. It takes practice to develop a comfortable physical routine, and the newborn may emit piercing shrieks when he's disturbed. New parents are challenged by the need to respond patiently and kindly—again and again—as they themselves become sleep-deprived and weary. Developing skills in handling their infant will help parents become confident in this new full-time job.

First-time parents are frequently uneducated in newborn care prior to having a baby, and find themselves faced each day with issues of diapering, dressing, bathing, soothing, holding, and feeding. Often they are amazed by how difficult such apparently simple things can be. They are grateful for offers of assistance, and may watch closely to see how someone with experience gets that shirt over baby's head, cleans her creases and folds, or gently soothes her to sleep.

I personally strive to model tenderness and respect for the newborn's experience. I remind the parents that the baby has gone through the tremendously difficult process of birth, as has the mother, and may be feeling quite uncomfortable in his body. I encourage them to observe him closely, learning his hunger signals, his need-to-burp cues, his signs of a bowel movement coming, the fussiness that precedes sleep. Most parents begin to understand the subtleties of their infant's

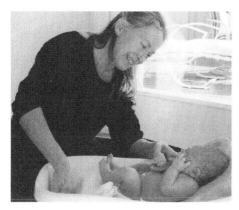

When the caregiver is calm, the infant feels secure —Photo credit: Julie Carter Hinson

behaviors quickly, especially when encouraged to pay attention to body language and the quality of the cry. I am happily impressed when a mother explains to me what her infant is expressing.

I speak calmly and warmly to the baby, and treat him as an honored guest. I try to help him to slowly adapt to his new surroundings, recognizing that our homes are filled with visual, auditory, tactile, and olfactory sensations. He may easily become over-stimulated and anxious. Dimming the lights, closing the door, turning off the phone and television can assist him to relax and sleep. Newborns require up to twenty hours of sleep each day, and are most content when this need is met. The common idea that keeping him awake during the day will cause him to sleep through the night is incorrect, as his natural rhythm requires frequent feedings followed by sleep, throughout all hours. A baby who is not allowed to sleep when tired will become very fussy. A well-rested baby rests well. I often remind parents of this truth.

While changing diapers and clothes, I speak quietly, and try to keep the baby warm. He doesn't need to be stripped down and left naked. This stimulates his anxiety reflex; arms and legs shoot out,

How to Soothe a Fussy Baby

It can be helpful to demonstrate a simple technique to calm a baby. This is one anybody can master, and it's amazingly effective!

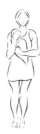 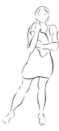 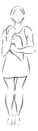

Hold the infant comfortably in arms. Standing erect, feet together, step to the right with right foot, then bring left foot to meet right (step, together).

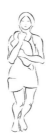 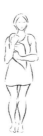

Bend knees to a comfortable level, then straighten (down, up)

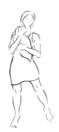 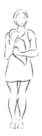

Step left foot to the left, bring right foot to meet it (step, together)

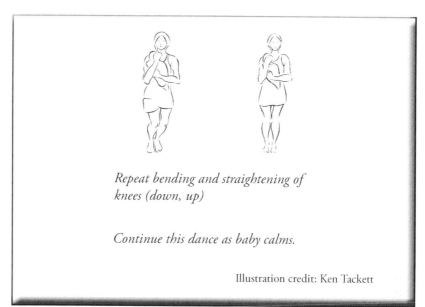

Repeat bending and straightening of knees (down, up)

Continue this dance as baby calms.

Illustration credit: Ken Tackett

waving uncontrollably, and crying begins. Instead, we can cover his torso with a light blanket, perhaps tucking in the edges to create a light swaddle as we clean the diaper area. When bathing the baby, we scoop warm water over his upper body, keeping him warm all over. Holding his arms or hands helps him feel secure. When the caregiver becomes anxious or hurried, the infant picks up on the feeling and becomes distressed, too. Staying calm is key. The doula can demonstrate this repeatedly.

The ability to soothe a fussy child may be the most coveted of all postpartum parenting skills! When a parent becomes proficient in this, confidence soars. There is a way of tuning in to the infant's body language, paying attention with a willingness to move and shift, rock and pat, until the child comes to rest.

The doula can demonstrate this over and over, maybe explaining verbally what she's doing and why. Let gravity help you and baby both. Place her against your chest, pat her back, and move rhythmically with a definite pulse. Every doula will want to develop excellent baby-soothing skills, demonstrating to parents that it can be done. What we want to model here is that infants do not need to cry a lot; that they are communicating a need of some kind. The need can usually be met, and they, the parents, can learn to respond successfully.

> *Having you in my home has shown me what a mother should do for her family. I have learned so much from you, and enjoyed every minute…*
>
> —Vickie, mother of three

Above all, we doulas are modeling our attitude. Because we are professionals, parents may see us as experts. How we handle the infant, speak to her and respond to her, may become the inner picture held by the parent, the perceived ideal. This is a huge responsibility.

Non-professional caregivers, friends and family members, also exert a big influence on new parents by their tone and behavior toward the child. Treat the baby gently, like the treasure that he is. You can help to set the stage for harmony in the family by acknowledging the special needs of each member and maintaining an attitude of compassionate service.

Chapter 6

SUPPORTING THE POSTPARTUM FATHER

I knew from the experiences of my four sisters that the hardest time in the adjustment to parenthood would be right after the birth. I sensed that Connie would need more care than I could give her, and we agreed to hire a doula. Her presence gave me a break from being a constant caregiver, a role I wasn't that comfortable with. As hard as the whole transition is for the mother, it's hard for the father too. As much as he wants to be involved, he feels a little separated at first. Our doula offered me a lot of support, too.

—Mark, first-time father

We are extremely grateful and appreciative of the assistance you gave us through this period of transition. You helped to provide some stability and center in our home which at times seemed to have more fear and turmoil. You allowed me to comfortably return to work and maintain my focus there during the day, knowing that things were under some "control" at home. You will certainly be missed. At the same time, we all feel much more capable and confident in our ability to manage and grow without you here.

—Cliff, M.D. and father of two

Men feel the pressure of a "new mouth to feed" in many ways. Their partners appear vulnerable, and in need of protection and care. The new baby is an enigma, and can be difficult to satisfy. The laundry and dishes pile up, messes go untouched. The expectations on the father may seem enormous, and he is not getting much sleep. Frequently, a man's employer allows him a week, maybe two, to stay at home after the birth. Unfortunately, that time goes by very fast, and it is several more weeks before things feel settled in the home. There is a period when the postpartum father may feel stretched thin, overextended, exhausted, trying to care for his wife and children, and working full time.

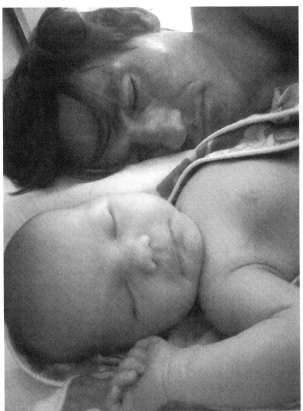

Napping with the baby is a good way to catch up on lost sleep —Photo credit: Kelly Born

This is where the doula can be tremendously helpful: catching up on tasks around the home, leaving dinner cooked and the table set, the sheets clean, toys picked up, children happy, mother rested, baby cozy and clean. When the new father enters his home after a day's work, it feels harmonious and welcoming. Things are in order, and best of all, his wife is content, calm, and nurtured. The doula has taken over the essential chores, so the mother can luxuriate in the mystery of new life, and can share it with her partner.

For first-time dads, learning to handle the baby is a challenge. They are often called upon to soothe a fussy baby, to perform a diaper change in the middle of the night, or to attempt to burp the infant. With no prior experience, this can be daunting. My role is to tenderly model baby-care techniques for the parents. As they see that the child calms down in my arms, they try to copy what I do. As they notice the baby doesn't cry when I'm changing his diaper, they watch to see my style and what I'm doing differently from them. One young father recently announced, "Everything I know about caring for my son, I learned from watching you!"

As a professional, I am a safe person to question, to listen to. We have no prior history; I have no agenda beyond helping to make the postpartum time pleasurable and healthful. There is no shame in admitting one's fears, worries, and lack of experience, but many fathers have no one to share their thoughts with. A caring and open-hearted doula is a good listener and a great source of knowledge. It's very important to nurture that relationship if the opportunity is there. An actively involved dad is priceless, and as his confidence in his abilities increases, so will his participation in the care of his child.

Each father is unique. Some I see each day; others I never see again after the prenatal visit. The big variable is his work schedule. If he leaves the house by 7 a.m. to commute to his job, returning 12 hours later, he needs me to accomplish as many household chores as possible, leaving the mother rested and restored, ready to be his loving partner, to enjoy their new baby with him. If, on the other hand, he works at home, his need may be to have some uninterrupted work hours behind closed doors; or perhaps time to leave home to do the errands or get some exercise.

Frequently, the reality is somewhere in between. Some men have flexibility in the mornings, to stay around and get the children off to school, for example, or to care for baby while mom gets a couple of hours of uninterrupted sleep in the early morning, when baby might be awake and playful. Others can leave work for an hour to pick up a preschooler or drive a child to an activity. Other fathers can arrange to work from home a day or two each week, being more available to their families' immediate needs. Each new dad must explore his options, and try to make his job as family-friendly as possible. I firmly believe that a happy family life affects an adult's performance in the world in a very positive way, and employers are benefited in the long run by understanding the needs of parents and children.

A few dads have shared with me over the years that it really helps their wives to have a woman to talk to. Of course this is true. It takes some of the pressure off the husband if the wife's emotions have had some expression, some release, during her time with her doula or her female friends. Men may be baffled by the hormonal roller coaster of our female reality, and postpartum is no exception. I have heard husbands complain of being unappreciated, unable to please their wives, "I can't seem to do anything right!" In my role as doula, I can see each person's point of view, and can help them to understand one another. Sense of humor is key here. Keep it light. Remember Mars and Venus, that men and women are innately different.

During the prenatal interview, I listen closely to the partner for cues as to what his real needs are. One man spoke at length about his wife's struggles after the birth of their first child. The baby was colicky and demanding, and the mother cried frequently and felt inadequate. Now this boy was an energetic four-year-old. I could hear that they were expecting a similarly difficult postpartum this time around. The woman's softness, her vulnerability and anxiety were evident. She felt she would "fail" again to be the perfect mother, and her husband would again be powerless to soothe her fears. I told them that I could see no reason at all to assume this baby would be colicky or high-need; it is not the norm. Each baby is entirely different in temperament, and we can as easily expect a perfectly calm child. There was a palpable shift in the air after I said those words, as if a tiny opening of hope and possibility had occurred for them.

After the birth, this mother and I bonded through talks and hugs as she shared her concerns and feelings. She took long naps while I held her peaceful daughter. Her mood stayed positive as long as she had the space to care for her own basic needs. After her little boy came home from preschool, I cared for the baby while mother and son had precious time together to take a walk, and then read stories while cuddling on the couch. Usually when the father arrived home from work, mother and children were happy and rested, and dinner was being prepared. The energy inside the home was entirely different from their previous experience, and it was a tremendous relief for the father. By the way, their baby girl was relaxed, calm, and beautiful, and was smiling by four or five weeks of age. She won my Happy Baby of the Year award!

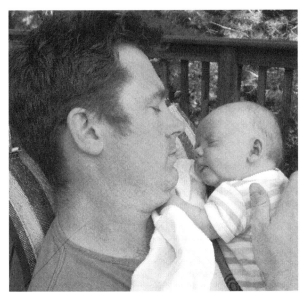

*Participating in baby care from the very beginning
allows a young father to bond deeply with his son and
create a parenting partnership with his wife* —Photo
credit: Sandi MacLeod

Sometimes the father's need revolves mainly around care of the
home. Especially if there are several children already in the family,
when the mother stops doing all the chores, things pile up fast! Dirty
laundry accumulates at an alarming rate, and is rather easy for the
doula or friend to help with by keeping the machines working. The
kitchen is vital, and I always leave it clean. Otherwise, it will become
dad's problem.

> *After one lovely mother gave birth to her fourth child by
> c-section, she came home from the hospital with an infected
> incision and a sick baby. Her ten-year old was in school and
> very self-reliant. The two- and three-year-old girls, one with a
> handicap, were at home. I spent many hours there. I stayed until
> dad walked in the door. Dinner was prepared, mom was rested,*

and the house was tidy. The little girls were bathed and dressed for bed, after we had laughed and sung our way through the afternoon playing on the swings and sandbox. In her letter to me, the mother shared how uplifting it was for her husband to come home to this happy family and clean home. "He was able to enjoy ME," she said, "because he wasn't needed to do everything else."

The doula can really assist the new father in getting involved in infant care. If this is new territory for him, demonstrate understanding and start with the basics. Show him how to hold his child, place her in his arms and drape a blanket over her to create a nest. Teach him how to bundle the baby onto his chest. Encourage closeness and tenderness. Sometimes dads want to show how tough their baby is, and may startle the child into an upset by handling her roughly at too tender an age. Others seem to fear their baby is breakable. In any case, the doula, as a professional, can share techniques, ideas and knowledge with fathers. It's our job, and often they will listen gratefully.

When my friend's wife gave birth to their first child, I stopped in to visit. I found Paul with a screaming infant. He was holding her at arm's length, bouncing her on his knee as fast as he could, with a look on his face that said, "Help!" I scooped up the baby and drew her in close to my body, supporting her head with one hand and covering her with a blanket, creating a cocoon of safety and warmth. She immediately relaxed and became calm. I began to sway gently, keeping her body against mine, as she settled into rest. Paul stared, open-mouthed, bleary-eyed, and exhausted. "Oh, thank you," he mumbled as he slumped back into the chair.

Without appearing condescending, we may offer our assistance, perhaps to soothe the child's crying or to change the diaper. We can model soft speech and gentle touch. When diapering, we keep the baby warm and calm, showing that the child doesn't need to scream through each diaper change. We can describe burping techniques, and how to recognize signs of digestive distress. We can listen to a father's worries about his wife, and reassure him that all will be well. Perhaps we can help him to understand her, and to suggest ways that he can support her. I frequently ask a husband to please be sure that his wife has a glass of water by her side when nursing, and remind him to feed her often. I engage him as part of the caregiving team, helping to provide purpose and inclusiveness. It's too easy for a father to feel pushed out of the circle of women. We must help his wife to kindly include him as he learns about his new role.

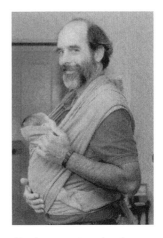

Dads can enjoy the closeness and ease of "wearing" the baby —Photo credit: Fatima Kazimi

I can't over-emphasize the importance of knowing how to soothe a crying baby. Many parents have joked to me about the baby-bounce that my body goes into when holding an infant. "If I could bottle that and sell it … !" They tell me of practicing the movement in the wee hours. Gentle rhythm and patting, moving up and down while gliding side-to-side, that's my style. You may have your own. Share it. A husband who can soothe his crying infant earns his wife's devotion and the respect of his peers.

Fathers and partners of birthing women have an opportunity to participate and enjoy the process of nurturing new life and parenting. Confidence and skill enhance this possibility, making the partner useful and successful in both baby- and mother-care. The doula or support person may tune in to the father's experience and gently assist him to develop the skills he needs. We also care for the family when he is away, offering a sense of security, and leaving a welcoming environment for his return. As with so many aspects of our work, what we do can make the difference between just getting through the day and enjoying what the day has to offer. This can be a transformational time in the life of the couple, and as caregivers we are in a position to help set the stage for positive shared experiences.

Chapter 7

SIBLINGS AND THE NEWBORN

Becoming an elder sibling to a newborn represents a tremendous change in a child's life. Up until now, he may have been the center of the family. From the perspective of the child's life experience, the awareness of both parents has been consistently focused on him. He is secure in his ownership of the affections of these two dependable adults.

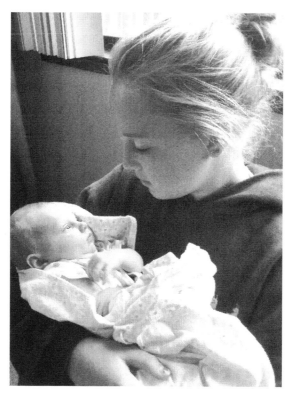

Connecting with a newborn is a profound experience for an older child —Photo credit: Lilia Webber

When the infant arrives on the scene, the focus will shift. Now the tiny newborn needs tender care, and big brother is seen as so independent and capable in comparison. He may be asked to be quiet, to wash his hands before touching the baby, to stay off the bed, to hold back from expecting mommy and daddy's constant care. He may hear, "No!" more often, and be taken off his mother's lap to make room for the nursling. He will have to wait his turn and accept changes in his routines. Perhaps the harshest cut of all is watching mommy coo and caress the sweet newborn. Soon the child realizes that the baby seems to be always in her arms! Frequently the older sibling will enjoy the baby's presence for a while, and then ask, "When will she go back? I'm ready for her to go now."

Newborns are irresistibly soft and cute, and toddlers love to touch their little hands, feet, and faces. Chubby fingers point out eyes and noses and stick into ears, often more roughly than we would like. We must carefully protect the infant from his sibling's ardor, while encouraging the demonstrations of affection. Children frequently squeeze the baby's hand or cheek too tightly, or press their own bodies against the baby's with more force than appropriate, seeming to hold a powerful and conflicting energy toward the infant, an energy that confuses them as well as us. Babies are tougher than they appear, but can be hurt by a zealous sibling. It is wise to leave the baby out of reach of older children, except when directly supervised. The older ones can be assisted to hold the baby in their lap, on a chair or couch, with pillows around and an adult hand close by. This is thrilling for the toddler, who is soon ready to move on to something more active.

The reactions of big brothers and sisters to a new baby are varied, but in most cases there is some kind of change in behavior. It may be an increased sensitivity, falling apart easily, or becoming frustrated

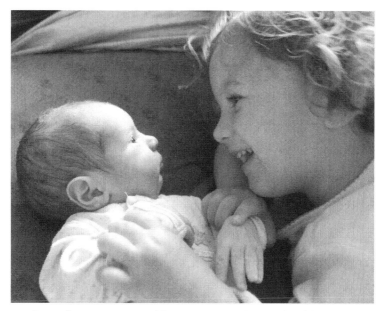

Little newborns are irresistible to curious and excited toddlers —Photo credit: Lisa Peevers

quickly. Sometimes it's temper tantrums and unreasonably angry behavior. There may be regression in potty training.

> *Luke was a very bright 4 year old who told me details about the origin of the universe. But shortly after the birth of his sister he pooped in his pants in preschool. Everyone was surprised, given his maturity and sophistication. He did the same for two more days. Luke's mother Valerie was concerned; this was becoming a problem for his caregivers. She gently reminded him that babies and small children wear diapers because they don't poop in the toilet, and offered him the option of a diaper. He considered this, and the next day returned to his use of the potty! Valerie handled it with understanding and respect, leaving Luke with no sense of shame.*

Two-year-old Lily, who had been completely out of diapers for several months, began to urinate wherever she was standing after her brother Ben was born. Sometimes when we were gathered in the living room Lily would suddenly announce, "I'm peeing!" as she watched the warm liquid run onto the carpet.

Usually a gentle and kind child, two-year-old Rhonda became very angry at her mother after the difficult birth of her baby brother. Her mother, Christina, needed to remain in bed for several weeks to recover from loss of blood and other complications. Her daughter refused to snuggle with her, and maintained a hostile attitude toward both her mom and her new brother. Christina was heartbroken, feeling helpless and unable to connect with her child. One day Rhonda picked up a shoe and smacked the baby in the head with it. This very difficult behavior went on for quite a few weeks, until mama was fully back to health and vitality, and little Rhonda was finally accustomed to the baby's presence. Meanwhile, she spent most of her time with her daddy, who fortunately was available and willing.

Some siblings seem to glide through the adjustment period without upset. However, parents should be aware and prepared to be understanding and compassionate if challenges arise. Keep in mind that this is probably the biggest change this child has experienced in his life thus far, and it may send his emotions on a wild ride. He needs to be reminded again and again that his world is still as secure and loving as always. His family is now larger, and he is now sharing the center of the circle, and all is well. It may take a while for him to accept this new reality.

As the caregiver, you can help by being a supportive and dependable friend to him. You can fix his food, read him stories, and help pick up his toys. Together you can fold laundry, load the dishwasher, or water the plants outdoors. You can go on outings, do errands together, take walks, and supervise play dates. Baking cookies, making cards for others, picking flowers for mommy's bouquet, or decorating baby's changing table are fun projects that encourage kindness to others.

I try to speak positively, with expectations of enjoyment, to create a happy space for the child. I want to be a special friend that is connected with the idea of the new baby, leaving happy memories and associations. I try to honor the child's reality, and help him to have fun. I'm not the disciplinarian, though sometimes I must be; I rather prefer to be the loving and playful auntie that everyone's happy to see.

Over the years I've learned how to play with little children, which I was usually too busy to do with my own. They love it when I sit on the floor and play dolls or trucks, or draw pictures, or create fantasy worlds with stuffed animals. I get right to their level, and we become fast friends. One thing I've learned about kids is their love of repetition. They want to repeat yesterday's game just as it was and then again tomorrow! One lovely little girl shared her favorite puzzle with me. The following day, she pulled it out again. At one point she expected a certain response from me, and I forgot how it went. I said the wrong thing, and she put her little head on the floor and cried! This was a big learning experience for me.

Young children often want to help, and enthusiastically join me in putting clothes in the washer, piece by piece, often identifying each item's owner; or washing dishes in the sink, perhaps with a little extra mess, but well worth it. They enjoy assisting in sorting clean laundry, and can help the doula know what belongs to whom. Sweeping, watering plants, and fetching items for mom or baby are all activities that small children can enjoy. Pulling a step-stool up to the changing table so big sister can participate in baby-care is a good way to make her feel included and important. Talk with her about what you are doing, and help her to get involved with baby.

In families that have several children, there will be a lot of housework for the doula to do, and as well, she will want to support the mother and baby by tending to the older children's needs. This can be a juggling act, much like motherhood, and it requires a willing and focused attitude. Sometimes the children will just want a playmate, and it seems impossible to get the chores done. Or the siblings will squabble, causing the doula to become the arbitrator. On occasion, the doula herself may become the scapegoat of a child's frustration. It is vital to maintain a loving presence, do the best you can, and remember that happy children are more important than a clean house.

Older children need to maintain their on-going activities after the first week or two of the baby's arrival. They will get bored or irritable around the parents' preoccupation with the newborn and the changed energy level in the home. It honors their individuality and importance to continue prioritizing their activities when possible. Doulas, dads, family friends, and playmates' moms can all help with this. Taking them outdoors to play, walk, run on the beach, or create games in nature is healthful for the children and makes a quiet house for mom and baby. Engaging children in calm indoor activities and attending to their ongoing need for attention is also helpful in the postpartum family.

A professional doula will want to determine her personal policy on driving children in her own vehicle, or in the family's car. It can be very helpful if the doula is available for school pick-ups or to take kids to the park or library, swim classes or dance lessons. Sometimes doing the family errands together is appropriate. If there are car seats, the parents may prefer the doula to drive the family car. It is important that the doula feel comfortable with this, and it's also OK to say no. Each doula and each family have their personal values, and decisions such as this should be worked out in the prenatal interview. Insurance and safety issues need to be considered.

Another vital way to support the elder sibling is to provide opportunities for her to be with her mom. I often will take the baby into my care, to allow the mother to give her full attention to her first-born. This precious relationship needs nurturing during this tender transition. I've heard many a mother bemoan the loss of the intimacy she shared exclusively with her older child, now that someone new is in her arms. An intuitive doula will pay attention to timing and moods, and encourage positive experiences of reconnecting. A few minutes of private time snuggling in bed with mom can work miracles for a grumpy two-year old.

Also important is to encourage the child's loving attitude toward the new baby. This is not done by forcing the issue, but by including the child in "ownership" of this new person. Let him participate. Invite his help by asking him to bring a diaper or pick out an outfit. If he is able, ask him to carry food or water to his mom. Show him what you're doing and what the baby needs. Remind him of how much he will teach this child. Encourage tenderness and caring by speaking softly and handling the newborn gently, using terms like "love" and "family" and "happiness" as much as possible.

It can be an automatic response to shout, "No!" if an older child is rough or inappropriate with a small baby. I remember one under-two-year-old boy who began to leap onto his twin siblings as they slept. I caught him in mid-air and exclaimed, "There are babies down there!" We laughed and became fast friends. Remember that children are watching our reactions to their behaviors. We want our responses to assure the child that we are friendly, safe, and supportive. It's such a relief to a tired mother to see her preschooler delighted to spend time with the doula, knowing that the child's age and sensitivity will be honored.

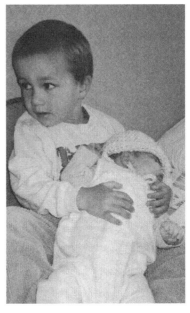

Siblings enjoy holding the baby for a minute or two —Photo credit: Lilia Webber

Early life experiences, though often forgotten, impact the future. We can help to set the stage for family harmony and sibling unity by meeting the basic practical needs of young children, providing the attention they require, feeding, bathing and playing with them, helping them stay balanced. We can keep their mothers comfortable and rested. When we care for the new baby, we provide the sibling private access to his mom. Happy memories of early life with a new brother or sister will encourage ongoing positive interactions and a warm relationship. Small but thoughtful acts on the part of the friendly caregiver or professional doula can pave the way.

Chapter 8

TWINS

You made such a huge difference in the first three months of Josh and Ian's lives. So many times I was completely overwhelmed by caring for twins and you showed me a nice, calm way to nurture and love them. You have a beautiful way with babies and their moms.

—Jane's letter to her doula

I miss you tremendously. You took such good care of me, taught me so much, and took such good care of the babies too. I'll never forget how you rocked my babies, gave me fruit, rubbed my feet and let me go on and on. I needed it so much.

—Marilyn, mother of twins

Several mothers of twins have said to me, "It must be really easy to have just one baby!" While that's not really true, twins present a challenge of fortitude and perseverance unlike anything else. The challenges of multiples beyond twins increase exponentially. In this chapter when I refer to "twins," I include other multiples. Yet, with each additional baby, new responsibilities and challenges present themselves, different techniques may be employed, and more care-givers are needed.

Twins are far more common than triplets, quadruplets, quin-tuplets, and beyond, and I base my remarks on my experience with many twins and their families. With a large number of couples using the technique of in-vitro fertilization to overcome fertility problems, many sets of twins are being born, and frequently to older parents. When twins are expected, parents are wise to line up dependable help in advance. The new mother will need round-the-clock support for at least the first couple of weeks. Hiring an experienced doula is an excellent way to complement the family members and friends who may be available to help out.

The miracle of twins brings with it a huge amount of chores, especially in the early months. Two individuals whose needs and temperaments vary, often widely, twin babies are a constant source of amazement, while requiring a continual stream of feedings and diaper changes. Carrying and bearing multiples is added strain on a woman's body, and often results in delivery by c-section, so the mother's need for rest and healing is significant. The new parents will be on duty 24 hours a day, and are greatly helped by opportunities to nap, shower, eat, etc. If the twins or multiples are the couple's first children, they will need additional assistance with getting to know and understand the needs of infants, and modeling of how to meet those needs.

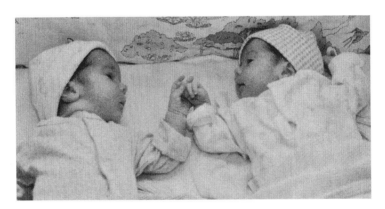

Twins, accustomed to each other's presence, often seem to prefer to sleep together—Photo credit: Fatima Kazimi

FEEDING FOR TWO

If the twins are preemies, depending on their level of prematurity, they may have difficulty latching on to the breast until their sucking muscles become sufficiently developed. If hospitalized, they may be fed formula, or if the mother pumps her breasts, colostrum followed by breast milk from a bottle, cup, or feeding tube. Mothers who want to nurse their hospitalized twins should pump regularly, keeping their supply up until they can nurse on their own. At home, the doula can help with the logistics of washing pump parts and bottles, preparing for the next round, burping babies, and assisting with any necessary supplemental feedings as well as regular attempts at latching-on to the breast. She can provide warm compresses to prepare the breasts for pumping or feeding. Often the twins are tiny and sleepy for a week or two, especially if they were preterm or late preterm. Mostly eating and sleeping, they give their parents a "grace period" to rest and recuperate until they begin to awaken to the sensations of existence. Weight gain is important at this time, and tiny babies may need to be aroused to be fed at regular intervals, generally every two to three hours, or more often.

Many parents decide to feed both babies on the same schedule, waking the second when one is hungry, to avoid a never-ending cycle of feeding. Some swear this is what keeps them from going crazy. On the other hand, some parents prefer to feed the twins separately, providing individual time with each baby. Others are entirely on-demand. Whatever works for the couple works for me.

Mothers of multiples can produce sufficient quantities of breast milk if the intention is strong and there are no extenuating circumstances. If both babies cannot feed at the breast, a breast pump can be employed to maintain her milk production and provide a steady supply of milk that can be offered via bottle, syringe, cup, or other vessel when the mother is nursing the other child. Feeding and pumping will take up a lot of the mother's time, so we assist her whenever possible by changing diapers during feedings, cleaning and preparing pump parts, taking over as soon as her job is finished. The need for a break each day is especially important to mothers of multiples, and naps are vital to mental and physical maintenance.

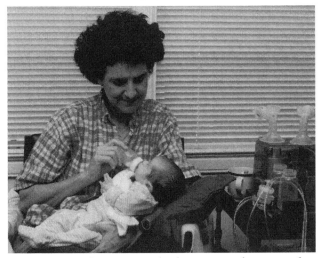

Some parents of twins or multiples use a combination of breastfeeding, pumping, and bottle-feeding —Photo credit: Frederick Yukic

Janie was determined to feed her twins exclusively with breast milk. She rented an electric pump and set it up on her lovely glass dining table. The middle of the night would find her here, pumping milk in the dark. There was always a supply of refrigerated milk to bottle feed one twin while the other nursed. It was hard, those first six months before solid foods were introduced, but she kept her commitment and those girls never tasted a drop of formula.

Breastfeeding two at once is certainly possible. A tandem nursing pillow makes a comfortable base for nursing twins. Help the mother prepare her nursing station with drinking water, spit-up cloths, and whatever else she needs. Put the pillow around her, then bring one baby at a time and assist in getting him latched on. The football hold is a popular way to hold two nursing babies, but when very little, cross-cradle hold works too. After the first baby is sucking, bring the second and get him going. Sometimes one will fall off the breast as the other is getting on, and it can take a few minutes of adjusting and readjusting to finally have them nursing together. The mother needs to have a helper to facilitate this balancing act until it gets easier, as the babies become habituated to nursing and develop muscle strength and coordination.

I have had women tell me they can't stand the stimulation of being suckled by two at once. These moms may prefer to take the time to nurse each twin alone, sharing special moments with each one. Sometimes they will ask another person to feed one twin with a bottle, syringe, or cup of pumped milk or formula if the babies want to eat simultaneously. Many twins become very versatile with using breast or bottle interchangeably. Of course, the more breast milk the better, and we encourage and support our moms in maximizing milk production; every set of parents will have their own ideas and preferences. Many moms of twins desire to share the responsibility of feeding with the other parent, friends or relatives, and so will routinely provide a bottle. Some feel they can't produce enough, and will supplement the babies at alternate feedings with bottles of formula to keep up with the demand. We respect each couple's decision and support them in finding the proper balance for their family.

Some twins are entirely formula-fed, especially if the newborns are hospitalized where there is limited support for breastfeeding. Some mothers after cesarean section are so groggy and uncomfortable that they don't want to try to nurse. While many Newborn Intensive Care Units encourage breastfeeding, some still may not due to space and staff limitations. If the mother desires to provide her body's nourishment to her babies, she can insist, and find ways to work with the nurses to fulfill this intention.

> *Carolyn never really wanted to breastfeed, but she agreed to the plan because it was her husband's preference. After she delivered her twins by undergoing a difficult c-section with significant blood loss, the thought of babies at her breast seemed impossible and overwhelming. Her distressed state was obvious to her husband, who gracefully stepped down from his position and supported her in doing what was right for her at the moment … bottle-feeding.*

This mom bonded well and became a wonderful, active and happy mother. Her children are bright, healthy and well adjusted. She did her family a service by honestly expressing what was right for her, and lovingly formula-feeding her infants. As her doula, I was in full support of her decision. I cared for both twins for a few hours each day while she slept, bathed, and attended to her own needs.

These and many other scenarios present themselves, and the doula works within each family's choices and styles. Products are available that prop bottles up for feedings so an adult is not needed to hold the bottle, and some parents use these, especially during the night. Such a device allows the infant to suck at her own pace. It can encourage snacking, however, rather than efficient and complete feedings. As the doula, I generally avoid using these, leaving them for the more challenging circumstances the parents come up against. Holding in arms if feeding just one, or face-to-face interactive feedings are my preference. The shortcuts are for overtaxed parents.

MANAGING TWINS

If the doula can successfully care for two babies at once, it is a great help to the parents. I have often used infant seats or car seats to prop babies up for feeding two at a time. I sit on the floor facing them or with my back against a couch or chair with one baby at each side. With a burp-cloth under each chin, I offer the bottles. Attentively, I observe their need for burp breaks, sometimes placing one over my leg while burping the other on my shoulder. A thick blanket on the floor can be another place to put one baby while attending to the other. A feeding may take an hour or more this way, but in the end everyone is full, burped, diapered, and ready to either sleep or happily interact with her surroundings.

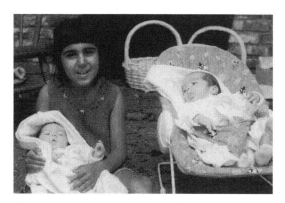

Keeping two infants happy is a big job! —Photo credit: Frederick Yukic

If one becomes fussy, I settle the other comfortably as I do the baby dance. Sometimes it's back and forth, settling one until the other fusses. Swings are helpful, as are infant seats, to help a baby rest. I can also hold two at once if necessary, especially with the help of a baby bundler or other carrier. The "wearing" of a baby is a wonderful way to have hands free to attend the other one, as well as providing close contact and security for the twin. Obviously, twins are often held less frequently than singletons, and wearing them is a great help. If the babies are crying, the parents won't rest, so we do our best to keep them content. When they are both asleep, we can start a load of laundry, prepare a meal or sweep the floor, but caring for the infants is the highest priority in families with multiples.

> *We were so lucky to be able to draw upon your experience,*
> *calm, and tranquility to help us, and we still don't know how you*
> *kept two infants calm, cleaned their clothes, and did the dishes*
> *all at the same time. We do think you had them under your spell!*
> —Darrel, father of twins

Chapter 9

SUPPORTING THE ADOPTING FAMILY

You saved us. We were so happy and tired and scared, and all the grandmas were unavailable. We waited so long for our baby to find us, there was so much heartache and disappointment along the way that we stopped reading baby books, stopped preparing. So when the time came and the baby came, I felt utterly inadequate and a bit lost. Unprepared for the extreme tiredness, terrified of dropping him or hurting him in some way. I am sure a lot of new parents feel these things. You made me feel safe, capable.

They say that the biggest psychological task for adopting parents is to really own it, to feel "entitled" to parent. I read that before our son was born and I thought it was silly. Of course I am entitled. Hah! It is truly an on-going issue, unless it is dealt with firmly, face-to-face. It is insidious, surprising. It is exacerbated by the silly and weird questions people ask you when you have an obvious adoption as we do, an interracial adoption. The most important thing you did for me is you validated me as a mom. I remember you kind of marveled at how hormonal I seemed. I had no way of knowing how the hormones feel to a new birth-mother, but it felt true when you said it and it gave me such hope and relief. I had a lot of fears going into this new role. I was conflicted and confused. Would I be a good mother? Would I be a "natural?" You helped me see that I was—you helped me relax into it, to enjoy his tininess, to honor his newness, and to surround him with love and safety. You helped me wrap him and tie him onto me and sway with him and sing to him. It's almost like a dream now, the love, joy, and tiredness: like we were on a baby cloud.

—Sage, first-time mother

Adopting parents are unique. Their process of bringing a child into their family is far different from that of birthparents, and they receive the baby without the physical experience of gestation and delivery. These natural events put a woman into a mental set determined by her biology; adopting parents come into the role through their desire partnered with willingness to go through the strife associated with the technicalities of adoption. Frequently they have been through heartache associated with failed pregnancies or attempts at pregnancy, or unsuccessful adoption experiences, and may be timid or afraid of further disappointment. We want to support them in embracing their new roles wholeheartedly, with expectations of joyful success ... indeed, they have succeeded, and the new reality has begun. They are now on equal footing with all parents of newborns; they will soon become sleep-deprived and focused on feedings and diapers, enchanted and perplexed by the tiny child in their care.

Sometimes babies come quickly to adopting parents, without much advance notice. I have worked with professional moms who need to complete projects or commitments before they can taper their work down to little or nothing. In these families, I have cared for the newborn while mom works, in an adjoining room or building, allowing frequent contact. Sometimes I have traveled with mother and baby to a workplace where the baby can remain close to the mother while in my care. These adjustments allow a new mom to feel responsible to the world she's leaving for now, while knowing that her baby is safe and content. Birthing women have nine months to prepare; adopting mothers often have far less. The need for a doula is increased by this lack of hormonal and practical preparation.

Alternately, some parents wait years for their baby, as Sage speaks

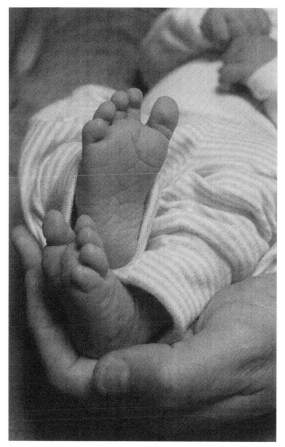

Adoption is an act of love in the giving and in the receiving —Photo credit: Maggie Muir

about in her letter. They may have begun to let go of the idea, or stopped reading and thinking about babies, and may be taken by surprise. They are frequently older and more settled, and the new routines insisted on by the infant can require a big adjustment, not always easy or comfortable. The doula can encourage them to slow down, take naps, limit their expectations of accomplishments beyond caring for the baby and themselves: eating, sleeping, bathing, that's about it in the beginning. Help them to honor the uniqueness of the moment, know that the child will never be like this again, and remind them of the preciousness of this phase of their parenting. This is the best opportunity to bond deeply with this treasured child; this is the time to begin to create a sense of trust and connection. They will find their rhythm, but first they must surrender to the change. We tidy their kitchens, prepare snacks, and cycle the laundry. We comment on the beauty of the child, and share their wonder. We answer their many questions, showing them the path of trusting themselves to parent and honoring their intuitive sense that has the answers they seek.

For a feeding experience that is closer to breastfeeding, some adopting moms choose to feed their baby with a supplemental nursing system. This device allows the baby to suck at the breast, while receiving milk or formula from a container via a tiny plastic tube attached alongside the nipple. It is satisfying and bonding for both mother and child, allowing skin-to-skin contact, eye gazing, and intimacy. The adopting moms in my experience who used this method consistently felt very satisfied and connected to their babies. It's not for everyone, though. The desire must be strong and the relationship aspect of breastfeeding valued.

Otherwise, the infant will be

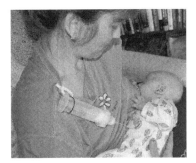

The Supplemental Nursing System allow the intimacy of suckling while providing fluid through a tiny tube —Photo credit: Salle Webber

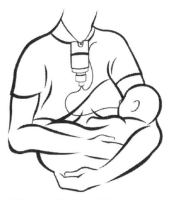

The Supplemental Nursing System — Illustration: Ken Tackett

bottle-fed. The parents may want to discuss the options of the various formulas available. By the time they're home with the baby, she may be a few days old and already feeding well. Be sure the parents have good bottle-feeding skills, holding at an angle, burping often, taking it slowly, with a cloth tucked under the chin for the inevitable leakage. Newborns generally consume one to two ounces at a feeding, working their way gradually to four ounces by about two months of age. Avoid overfeeding. Remember that a baby's stomach is smaller than her fist, so small, frequent feedings are best. Formula, because it is slower to digest, often keeps a baby feeling fuller for longer than breast milk does, so the adopted newborn may easily go three or more hours between feedings.

Possibly the most important role the doula plays in adoptive families is modeling the skills of infant care, and displaying a relaxed attitude toward parenting. These new parents are watching us for cues and understanding. They may be anxious and hormonally unprepared for this daunting task they've asked for, and we can help them to maintain a sense of humor and confidence as we show how to calm a crying child, how to wrap a baby in a bundler for a long nap, how to hold, burp, change a diaper, clean a crease. It is essential that we continually affirm how well they're doing, how content the child is, the signs of their growing understanding, and the apparent perfection of it all, their baby finding them and knowing them to be the perfect parents. I have seen little ones who seem so serene in their new environment, as if it was all their idea from the start!

Chapter 10

KEEPING COLLIN WHOLE

Shan was from Taiwan, and her English-speaking skills were minimal. Nevertheless, she worked beside her American husband, Vince, in their manufacturing business, and was clearly very bright and on top of things. As her doula, my ability to perceive what she needed was important, and our conversations were infused with pantomime and laughter.

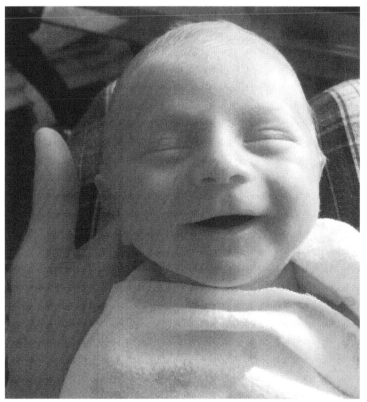

Glad to be born a boy! —Photo credit: Sarme Williams

One afternoon Vince asked me if I would accompany Shan to the pediatrician appointment the following day, as he couldn't get away from work. I readily agreed, and the next day I dressed baby Collin as Shan got herself ready to go out. We drove to the doctor's office, and upon entering, I was surprised to notice that the waiting room was empty. The receptionist called out, "Have you got the circumcision-consent forms ready?" Shan looked at me in bewilderment, and I, stunned, asked the woman, "Is that what we're here for?" Surprised at my question, she informed us that we were indeed scheduled for a circumcision.

I asked Shan, "Is this what you want?" She didn't understand; what does the word mean? I explained the procedure in the simplest terms, as her face took on an increasingly horrified expression. "Is this done to boys in your country?" I asked her. She shook her head emphatically, no. No! "Is this what my husband wants?" she inquired of me. I didn't know; but observing the mounting distress in Shan's face, I hardly cared. She had previously told me that she intended to spend time each year with her family in Taiwan, and I imagined this half-Anglo child playing with the local children, with his circumcised penis looking quite different from the rest.

I told the receptionist that we were sorry, but there had been a misunderstanding. We needed to discuss the subject with the baby's father, and would call if we wished to reschedule. "That's not possible," I was informed. The last day for this procedure to be done in the office was today. After the age of two weeks, the standard circumcision board, a piece of plastic with a cut-out shape of a baby's body and straps to hold down the straining infant, was considered no longer adequate, and Collin would have to be circumcised in the hospital. She was threatening us, I realized. Do it now or you'll be sorry!

But there's no turning back from circumcision. I tried to visualize Shan watching her baby be strapped down and cut, his screams piercing the air, and I knew I had to intervene. She didn't want this procedure; she was scared and confused. She was looking to me for guidance, for help answering this persistent woman who had stayed through her lunch hour for this appointment, to avoid other patients hearing the screams of the baby as his foreskin was surgically removed. The receptionist was irritated by our hesitation.

I took a deep breath and stood up. Shan quickly stood with me. I announced that we could not go through with this procedure without more clarity, that we regretted wasting the doctor's time, and would take responsibility for arranging a hospital circumcision if necessary. It was a communication problem, and Shan apologized as she rushed out of the office clutching her infant son.

She broke down in the car, her muted sobs expressing her fears of displeasing her American husband, along with her shock and horror at the thought of what had almost happened. I was relieved that the circumcision had been prevented, but anxious about Vince's reaction. Obviously, he knew what the appointment was for.

After we arrived at home, Shan went to bed, emotionally exhausted, and quickly fell asleep. The phone rang; it was Vince. "How did the pediatrician visit go?" he asked me. I took a deep breath, "Well," I began, and I carefully described the incident. "I'm very sorry, if it's what you wanted, but I was concerned for Shan."

There was a long pause. Vince's voice wavered as he spoke, "Thank you, thank you. I had no idea … I just assumed … I don't really think circumcision is necessary … but I showed her the paper and she said 'yes,' at least I thought she did, but she says that, you know, when she doesn't understand. Oh, this would have hurt her; thank you so much for protecting my wife!"

This was a happy ending to this chapter of Vince and Shan's parenting journey. Once the decision not to circumcise is made, it rarely comes up again. As a doula, focused on the well-being of the family, I am opposed to anything that unnecessarily causes distress or physical risk to a newborn. That's my job. I am convinced that circumcision does both.

I do discuss this issue with parents if appropriate, as I have found there to be a tremendous lack of education in this area. Unless parents specifically seek out alternative sources of information, there is not much advocacy within mainstream care for the right of a boy to an intact body. Though many doctors are no longer convinced of the necessity of circumcision, they rarely offer information to parents about the pros and cons, or what the procedure actually entails, but merely give them the choice to circumcise or not.

I choose to be more proactive in this area, encouraging parents to leave their son's body whole unless there is a compelling reason to do otherwise. Explaining the actual procedure step-by-step is often enough to cause parents to reconsider this "routine" surgery. Many people simply believe it's the right and necessary thing to do because it has been routine for so many years. It's what's done. In fact, it's what used to be done, and the trend is quickly turning. Parents need to hear this, need to know that if they do circumcise, their child may be the one that's "different" in the locker room a few years down the line. They need to hear of the risks of the surgery, the absence of medical reasons for it, and understand the sexual implications of circumcision for a baby who will probably spend the majority of his years as a sexually active man.

However, if a decision is made to circumcise, I am supportive of parents and child. I do my best to care for the baby gently, following directions for cleanliness during the period of healing and making him as comfortable as possible. I do not criticize the decision.

When the choice to circumcise is based on religious tradition, the parents may have conflicting feelings, as I have witnessed, but generally feel joyful to bring their son into the community through this ritual. The doula may be asked to be present, to care for the child after the ceremonial portion, when the guests are socializing and sharing food. Though I am not Jewish, I have occasionally been present for this purpose at the bris, a ceremony of circumcision and naming of the eight-day old infant. I have stayed in the background, ready to receive my charge at the appropriate time, to comfort and hold him for a couple of hours of deep sleep. Often the baby has been given wine-soaked fingers to suck on for comfort as his circumcision is performed. The parents are relieved to have a trusted caregiver for their infant while they fulfill their duties as hosts.

With love in her heart, the doula strives to support all members of the family, regardless of whether she would personally make the same choices they've made. We recognize that this is the beginning of a journey of many years, with choices to be made every day, and we continually work to support the development of parental self-confidence.

Chapter 11

VERONICA AND LAUREN

I parked the car in the driveway below the house, and took a moment to quiet my thoughts and prepare to enter the home of 50-year-old James, his wife Veronica, a first-time mom in her thirties, and Lauren, their baby girl. I had grown fond of this family since the birth four weeks earlier, and had spent most weekday afternoons with them. The sun warmed my face as I walked up the path, but I was jolted from my reverie by the screams of a hysterical infant. I hurried to the door and heard Veronica's angry voice. As I rushed into the room, she was shouting, "You can't control me! You need to stay where I put you! You're not in charge here!" She was leaning over the bassinet, red-faced and screaming, as her baby screamed back in terror. I reached for Lauren, and Veronica stopped me. "Don't pick her up! Don't you dare pick her up! She has to learn!"

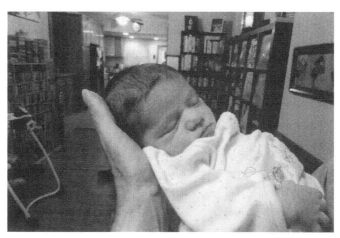

Babies are born into a complex world where much may be expected of them —Photo credit: Karen Rowe

I froze. Every molecule in my body strained toward this child, my every urge was to soothe and protect her. A baby's cry is a call for help, announcing something urgent and requiring prompt attention. Yet, I was bound to respect this mother's choices. I was there to support her, not to tell her what to do or how to parent her child.

Certainly, if she had been physically harming the baby, I would be morally and legally bound to step in. But she wasn't. She was merely allowing her infant to cry without comforting her. This is not considered criminal, and is unfortunately common behavior for many parents.

I turned to the sink, where Lauren's cries struck my back like whips. Allowing the warm water to run over my trembling hands, I breathed deeply. I longed to run away, but I couldn't abandon this distraught baby, or her mother. I put my hands to work in the sink, and gave myself a moment to calm my own tears and regain some semblance of strength and purpose.

From our hours together, I knew Veronica to be a loving and careful mother, attentive, striving to do everything "right" for her child. Perhaps her high self-expectations had pushed her over the edge. I remembered her goodness, her sensitivity and emotional fragility, and released my initial judgment of her behavior. I only wanted, at that moment, to make it better.

I followed Veronica into the other room, and gently touched her shoulder. She turned to me, leaned against me, weeping, and we held each other. As her body shook with sobs, I felt deep compassion for her, for all of us. Motherhood is demanding, overwhelming, and we are pushed to our limits and beyond. We've all been there. After a while, as her sobs began to subside, I whispered in her ear, "May I go and comfort Lauren please?" She nodded, yes, and rushed to her bedroom where she cried into her pillow, alone with her feelings of frustration and regret.

I held Lauren tenderly for a very long time. She fell asleep exhausted in my arms. Her mother, too, slept deeply, awakening later with a renewed intention toward patience, and a nagging sense of regret. I reassured her that all mothers, myself included, shared these struggles and moments of less-than-perfect parenting. We simply begin again with intention to do better next time.

Chapter 12

POSTPARTUM MOOD DISORDERS

Giving birth is a vivid and life-altering experience. The physical challenges and the emotional adjustments are huge. The body is exhausted from the exertions of labor, as well as the months of nourishing the infant within. Much fluid is lost, and the birthing woman becomes physically depleted. Her sleep cycles are continually interrupted by the needs of the newborn, and sleep deprivation sets in. The levels of stress hormones rise and the body's inflammatory response is triggered. High levels of inflammation contribute to mood swings, changes in appetite, sleep, sexual and social behaviors, all behaviors associated with depression. In turn, these behaviors contribute to increased inflammatory response, creating a potentially downward spiral (Kendall-Tackett, 2007).

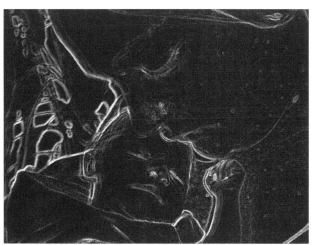

Emotional imbalance can significantly color the postpartum months —Photo credit: Joann Wilfert

BABY BLUES

Sometimes this combination of factors results in a mild form of depression, commonly called "baby blues." A new mom may alternate between laughing and crying, feeling extremely tender and insecure, or restless and irritable. In some cases a drop in thyroid function also occurs, causing fatigue, irritability, or lack of interest. She may feel like a failure, as she encounters the perplexities of breastfeeding and newborn care. How can we strengthen her? With warm, nourishing foods, fresh water, a clean bed, and frequent opportunities to nap. We care tenderly for her infant. The mother needs to know that she will be protected, and have companionship through this challenging adjustment. We encourage her to surrender to the rhythms of her newborn. Receiving devoted attention, a new mother will generally pass through this stage rather painlessly, as support, rest, and nourishment are the healing factors in her condition. In other words, postpartum doula care can prevent postpartum blues! Although reports say that up to 70 percent of postnatal women experience some form of depression or baby blues, I see very little of it because good care helps prevent it. One or more supportive and attentive friends coming by regularly can also help a new mom to maintain her emotional balance.

POSTPARTUM DEPRESSION

Beyond baby blues, which generally last up to two weeks, some women experience a more serious and longer lasting condition, known as postpartum depression. This may be characterized by prolonged periods of crying, withdrawal, inability to cope with the demands of the child, feeling angry at her mate and the baby. It may include poor appetite, inability to sleep, and lack of focus. It often occurs later than the baby blues, anytime within the first year, and tends to be more common in women who have experienced depression at other times in their lives, so it is wise to be prepared.

Studies have shown that breastfeeding encourages the lowering of stress hormones and inflammatory molecules, and promotes relaxation, suggesting that non-breastfeeding moms may be at a higher risk for depression. Excess pain from childbirth or surgery, or sore nipples while nursing can influence mood, as can past or present trauma, extreme sleep-deprivation and a lowered immune response with loss of vitality and physical well-being.

Again, the need to replenish body and spirit are the core factors. Feed the mother well, keep water nearby, provide a clean and welcoming place to rest, help her find time to nap, and above all, support her emotionally. Be there. Be available to listen, to care for the baby and provide her some time for herself. The sense of abandonment, being left alone for hours with a newborn, with no adult companionship, is detrimental to the delicate mental health of new moms. The doula or the attentive care-provider is the perfect person to fulfill these needs, as well as to encourage other family and friends to do the same when we're not there. Frequent and sincere affirmations of the wonderful work she's done, and continues to do, are important. She may be feeling inadequate to meet the seemingly endless demands of her new baby, so we may share stories that show her that we all felt that way, but survived and moved on to the next stage. I have found humor to be very effective in allowing a new mom to see her situation from a new perspective; to laugh, and see the joy and humanity in it, but sometimes mom and baby need space and a gentle touch to help them recover from a difficult birth and find their way.

Sarah was a delicate flower, both petite and emotionally fragile. Her expectations of birth and motherhood included pain and difficulty, with little confidence in her ability. Her husband was kind but easily overwhelmed by his wife's sensitivity. When their baby was born, Sarah's fears were realized with a hard labor ending in a c-section, and a baby requiring immediate medical attention. The first few days in the hospital were a challenge, with the newborn receiving what colostrum his mother could pump, and a delayed onset of milk production. Sarah was uncomfortable as her incision began to heal, cried frequently, and expressed feelings of inadequacy. She seemed to fear her infant, and held him with tension in her body. He didn't breastfeed easily, and Sarah was sure she had no milk. The hospital staff responded by feeding him with formula and encouraging the mother to sleep. Her anxiety increased and her mood fell deeper into darkness.

When the family finally went home, the doula encouraged skin-to-skin resting of mother and babe, exposure to the breast and frequent suckling. The new mother resisted, settling in to the idea that she couldn't provide what her baby needed. She was becoming resigned to the use of bottles of formula. The husband's support was enlisted, and the mother and child were tucked into their bed with all needs for food, fluid, companionship, and assistance met. The close proximity of the breast seemed to stimulate the infant, and the mother began giving more tender and confident attention to him. Husband and doula offered encouragement and affirmation. Over a period of two days of rest and bonding, Sarah's milk supply increased, the infant figured out how to use his mother's breast, and Sarah began to smile.

This began a successful breastfeeding experience, with Sarah expressing pleasure at her own nurturing abilities. With continuous support from those around her, Sarah maintained her emotional balance, avoiding the slip into depression that she had feared. Her body's natural response to her child provided the confidence she needed to move into her new role.

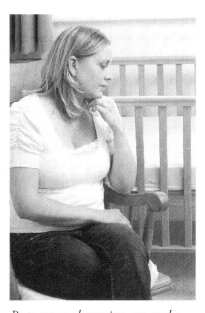

Postpartum depression can make every aspect of mothering more difficult and can affect how mothers feel about themselves, their partners, and their babies —Photo credit: Monkey Business

Other mothers may find that breastfeeding is too much to cope with while dealing with depression and will find alternative ways of feeding and caring for their babies.

Karen had spent most of her adult life in a mild state of depression, so she expected her postpartum to be miserable. Everyone said it would be. She knew the health benefits of breast milk, and was determined to provide this ideal food to her infant, but the idea of nursing was unattractive to her and she readily said so. The birth was an unplanned c-section, requiring mother and infant to remain in the hospital for several days. Because of the drowsy and depressive effects of surgical drugs and pain medication, breastfeeding got off to a rocky start. The nursing staff encouraged Karen to pump her breasts, and they bottle-fed her baby.

By the time the family came home, this pumping and bottling routine had become the norm. I urged Karen to put baby Jacob to her breast. He squirmed and fussed, refusing the soft breast and nipple, so different from the firm plastic of the artificial nipple. Karen's tolerance for frustration was soon reached, and she handed him to me and retreated to her room. I encouraged her to utilize techniques for firming the nipple, getting the milk flowing before offering Jacob the breast, tickling his lips to encourage opening, and to keep trying. Daily we tried, with always the same result. Karen would offer Jacob the breast, he would cry and wriggle, she would begin to cry, he would cry harder, and Karen would hand him to me and go to her room.

Soon Karen decided that she would pump as much milk as she could for six weeks. She quickly discovered that she could produce abundant amounts with more frequent pumping, and ultimately acquired a freezer supply that lasted a week after she stopped pumping.

Over time, and with cessation of lactation, Karen found her balance as a mother. She didn't want my companionship; she desired solitude. She found her own way. The part I played was to provide quality infant care so she could retreat fully into herself for several hours a day. I also did household tasks and some cooking, helping to make her home comfortable as she moved into her new reality.

As Jacob grew, Karen's confidence did too. When he was ready to add solid foods to his diet, mealtimes became more fun and less stressful. Karen's husband developed his skills and became a more participatory parent, allowing Karen some time for herself each day. As the months passed, the little family found its rhythm and developed working routines for ongoing daily life.

Karen's story reminds me that we must not have expectations about what is the right path for another person. We do our best to offer support and compassion, then step back and allow the process to unfold.

If a new mom continues to be depressed, it may be helpful or necessary for her to see a therapist for counseling. She may meet with a psychiatrist, who may prescribe antidepressant medication. If she is breastfeeding, it is vital that her doctor be selective in his choice of medications, prescribing from the available options one that is considered compatible with lactation. Moms who have weaned their infants to allow for antidepressants have often found themselves more depressed as they bottle-fed. The story of Ramona, in the chapter "Breastfeeding Support," illustrates this beautifully. If it is deemed necessary, a new mom can come through her depression with the aid of medication, allowing a more attentive and loving connection between mother and infant.

Essentially, how she is cared for in the weeks following delivery can make all the difference in her state of mind. I have seen this many times. Women often expect to be depressed. They have been unhappy at other times in their lives, and it's their programming. We can demonstrate compassion and understanding, provide beautiful plates of food, warm tea, offer baths and naps, and the hand of sisterhood. Truly, it can change everything.

POSTPARTUM BIPOLAR DISORDER WITH MANIA

Less frequent than depression, but potentially even more disruptive to family harmony, is bipolar disorder with mania. Bipolar disorder can occur with or without psychosis. In this disorder, mothers become hyperactive, hardly sleeping, working on unrelated projects with zeal and insistence, often ignoring the baby. They can be found in the wee hours, when the rest of the family is asleep, writing emails and composing blog entries, creating art or poetry, reorganizing closets, ironing clothes, or pacing the floor of the living room to avoid waking the others.

Generally, the mother reports that her head is reeling with ideas, and she feels filled with creativity that must be expressed. Unfortunately, the lack of sleep and mental agitation soon result in impatience and unreasonable demands on others. The mom may be unresponsive to the needs of her infant or other children. Her condition deteriorates with her continued lack of sleep and self-care. The medical care-provider should be notified immediately. Therapeutic or psychiatric intervention is almost always necessary. The stress of childbirth can trigger manic as well as depressive episodes. It can also occur when a mother is showing depressive symptoms and is treated with SSRI antidepressants, such as fluoxetine (Prozac). These medications can trigger a manic episode, helping to expose the underlying postpartum bipolar disorder.

Elaine was a bright and talented writer and mother with bipolar disorder. The first day after the birth of her second baby girl, she became manic. She found herself flooded with images and thoughts, she couldn't sleep, and felt no need to eat. By the third day, she had recognized herself as being in a manic state, and decided she must write a book on postpartum mania! She stayed up all night writing, feeling productive; she was providing a beacon for other moms. When I arrived to help the family on the fourth day she enthusiastically described this to me. Her body was beginning to crash from the extreme lack of rest and replenishment. This was the beginning of a challenging experience for me, and certainly for Elaine and her family. I spent many hours there, helping her to regulate her energy, urging her to rest, preparing food, and bringing the baby to her when she needed to be fed. I would specifically ask her to sit down and hold the baby for a while, which she loved but would forget to do. To help control her inappropriate busyness, we would laughingly say, "if you can't do it in a horizontal position, don't do it!"

Elaine went through bouts of therapy and psychiatry. She and her husband often fought bitterly, especially on weekends when there was no outside help. The level of guilt was high, as well as shame for allowing the children to witness these events. I spent lots of time befriending the older child, bringing stability into her days. The baby began receiving more and more formula, as the father took over more nighttime care, or others fed the baby when Elaine was in an agitated state. I found that my devoted attention to Elaine kept her generally calm, and she trusted and confided in me. However, outbursts frequently occurred in my absence, coloring the mood of the home the next day.

When mood-altering drugs were prescribed, new issues arose. They made her feel lethargic and dull, lacking all enthusiasm, but she didn't pick fights with anyone so they were seen as helpful. She tried many varieties of prescription drugs, and disliked them all. Elaine has investigated alternative remedies, herbal and nutritional, and has found results with these. She also has had relapses. Since she has bipolar disorder, hers may be a lifetime search for balance.

POSTPARTUM PSYCHOSIS

Infrequently, a new mother will demonstrate psychosis, in which case she may feel the urge to harm her baby or herself, or disassociate entirely. She may refuse to eat or care for herself or her infant. She may be hallucinating, seeing things others don't see, and exhibiting severe agitation or bizarre behavior. She may appear delusional one minute and lucid the next. This is an extreme and dangerous situation, requiring medical and psychiatric intervention. This condition is frequently seen with women who have bipolar disorder or forms of schizophrenia, but also often occurs for the first time after giving birth. If a doula finds herself with a psychotic mother, her first concern must be the safety of the infant, as she sends immediately for help. It is recommended that the mother be taken to the Emergency Department, keeping someone with her and the baby. Notify her care provider.

SUMMARY

Postpartum mood disorders are complex, and there are no pat answers. However, in my experience, if we can assist a woman to get over the first hump in her transition in a smooth and supported manner, she will be more likely to do well. If everything falls apart at the beginning of her mothering, and there is no one to pick up the pieces and lovingly help her to begin again, she may find mothering stressful and overwhelming. The first weeks postpartum are an investment in the family's future; contentment and confidence breed more of the same, as do frustration and feelings of inadequacy.

In cases of depression, some women may wish to investigate alternative therapies, in conjunction with an acupuncturist, naturopath, or nutritionist. Good results have been seen with the use of herbs, supplements, dietary adjustments, and bodywork. It has been well documented that omega-3 oils decrease inflammation, which can reduce the risk for depression. Mild exercise reduces stress and negative emotions. St. John's wort is an herbal antidepressant worthy of consideration. These and many other non-traditional therapies are available under the supervision of a qualified practitioner.

SECTION II

THE SKILLS OF CARE

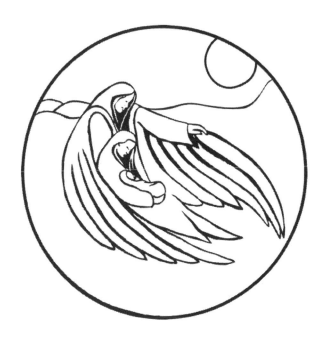

Chapter 13

CARE OF THE HOME AND FAMILY

The home becomes sacred ground with the entrance of a newborn. Its care may be seen as devotional necessity, and entered into with joyful willingness. This may seem grandiose when referring to piles of dirty dishes and laundry, unmade beds stained with bodily fluids, wet towels on the floor, toys strewn about; but this is where the mysteries of life unfold. This is the sanctuary where each family member can express him or herself in safety and comfort. The doula has the opportunity to quietly and calmly add the dimension of order to the situation by taking on small tidying tasks.

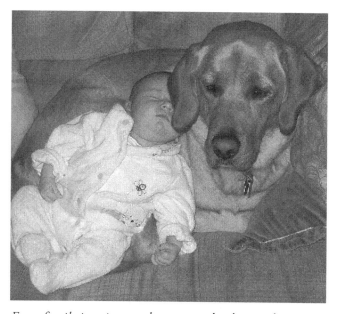

Every family is unique and every member has needs —Photo credit: Lindsey MacLeod

It is our goal to encourage the new mother to rest and enjoy her baby. This is most likely to occur if the daily household duties are attended to. She can relax as she looks around at a tidy home, not feeling a need to get up and clean or put something away. Sometimes, the husband or partner will take care of cooking and cleaning, but he, too, is missing out on sleep at night, and his life has turned upside down. It is a gift to him to offer help with the chores, wash the dishes, catch up on laundry, or prepare a meal.

KITCHEN CARE

The kitchen is probably the room most in need of attention. Emptying and loading the dishwasher, or washing dishes carefully in the sink, wiping counters, putting food away, and sweeping the floor are daily necessities. I pay close attention to putting things in their proper place, and I'm willing to ask what I need to know. It's not helpful to put items in the wrong place. I once was helping a new mom choose an ongoing caregiver. She invited a potential helper over, asking me to "train" her. As we worked together in the kitchen, I observed that as this helper was putting clean dishes away, she saw that the cup shelf seemed full. Instead of moving things around to make enough space for the clean cups, she simply put them somewhere else. This was inappropriate. It is not our job to make life confusing or frustrating for the new family. Caring for tiny details is partly what makes our work so valuable. As I wiped the coffee stains from a washed cup, one mom thanked me profusely for noticing such things. She said she is often aware, after I leave, of small things I've done for her that make a difference … a plant cleaned of dried leaves, crumbs removed from the innards of the toaster, a child's highchair wiped clean. In another home, I scrubbed the accumulation out of a container used to carry kitchen scraps to the backyard compost bin. The new mother so appreciated that I took the time to clean it thoroughly for her. Small things do mean a lot.

LAUNDRY

Laundry support is usually necessary in postpartum homes. I always discuss with a parent what their routines are ... cold or warm wash? What doesn't go in the dryer? Do they sort by color? Do they want to separate baby items from the others? It's necessary to respect how the particular family likes things done in order for them to feel comfortable turning tasks over to you. Remember to get the machines working for you early in your visit, to facilitate cycling a couple of loads while you're there. Try to wash, dry, fold and put away. If you're leaving things in the washer or dryer when you depart, be sure to let the parents know. It may be appropriate to put away the clean baby items, while leaving the parents' clothes in neat folded piles in the bedroom, unless you have been told specifically where things go. Some parents have more need of privacy than others, especially regarding the bedroom. This is an area you must "feel out" as the doula. Sensitivity to personal preferences is essential.

If there are small children in the family, there's likely to be lots of laundry. Getting as much done as possible is our goal. This is an area where younger children may be helpful; they can sort by color, put items in the machine with you, identify what belongs to whom, and show you where things go. This "help" may slow you down, but it engages the child in a positive way and will make you a better friend. It also allows the older child to feel helpful, responsible, more grown-up, and clearly different from the tiny, helpless newborn.

Sheets may need to be changed frequently, as mom is bleeding, milk is flowing, baby may spit up, and diapers can leak. I offer often to do this task, recognizing the need and understanding the comfort of clean sheets. The mother and infant are ideally spending a lot of time in bed, and we want it to be an appealing option. I like to make the bed neatly, then pull down the covers on the mom's side of the bed as an invitation to get in and relax.

HOME CARE

The bathroom used by the mother may require attention. If she plans to use the tub, be sure it is very clean. Her body is open and vulnerable to infection for up to six weeks after birth. The bathroom trash will fill with used sanitary napkins, baby wipes, disposable diapers, etc. Empty it often.

The cleanliness of floors makes a visual difference in the appearance of a room, so sweep the kitchen and offer to vacuum other areas. Pick up small things that are out of place. Fold blankets, fluff pillows, pile books and magazines neatly. If there are toys strewn around, put them in order. Do the things you would do in your own home as daily maintenance. Again, I repeat, don't be over-zealous and change things around. We want to support this family to feel comfortable with our help, to know we're part of their team, honoring their choices and style of living.

As a professional doula, I've found that there is a wide range of variation in the needs and expectations of parents regarding household support. This is an important area of discussion in the prenatal interview. Some families see me as the one who will clean up after them, while others prefer to keep my attention on the newborn. Some people have a weekly house cleaner that handles the heavy work, while others do not. I try to do what is needed … if the toilet needs cleaning, I clean it. If the mother is the one who usually does it all, I try to take over as much as I can. It is helpful to remember that all work is honorable, whether it is taking out the trash or holding the baby.

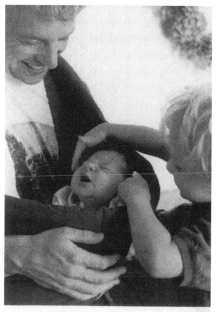

A confident dad enjoys his children as mom rests at home —Photo credit: Maggie Muir

Another area of support is with errands. Grocery shopping, picking up supplies at the local drug store, dropping off library books or outgoing mail, or even stopping by the used baby clothes shop for extra diaper wraps or sleepers … all these things and more may come up for the doula. I often tell families that they can call me prior to my arrival with a grocery list, and I'll shop before I come to the home. When I do this, I shop as carefully as if it were my own family's groceries, selecting individually every apple or plum or head of lettuce.

I ask the questions I need answered to do the job right: whole milk or low fat? How many bananas? What kind of bread does the family prefer? In some cases, the new mother may ask me to pick up sanitary supplies or something the baby needs, knowing that I understand what's needed, probably better than her husband does.

I have often been asked to water the houseplants or even the garden. A mother of newborn twins once said to me, "Either you've been watering the plants, or they just haven't died yet!" It was me. Another family had an apple orchard that was ready for harvest as the child was born. Daily, the mother asked me to go out and pick some apples: a few for the family to eat, some more to make an apple crisp, her favorite treat, as well as a bagful for me to take home to my own family. Have I mentioned the wonderful gratitude and generosity that I've been blessed with from the families I help? Often I return home with gifts and goodies.

Animal care, such as exercising the puppy, walking the dog, sweeping under the birdcage, making sure the cat doesn't get out, or checking food and water bowls, may be helpful in some postpartum homes. I have fed goats and chickens, collected eggs, and played with baby kittens. As a doula, I strive to be receptive to whatever the unique needs may be in every situation. And it's fun!

Sometimes there's a need for appointment support, especially after a c-section. New moms may not be ready to drive for a while, and may want me to go along as the driver and caregiver for the baby. Or they may prefer to leave the baby at home with me when they go to the doctor. If the appointment is with a dentist, a hair or nail salon, I encourage the mother to leave the baby at home, as the air in these environments may contain substances that are unhealthy for a newborn's delicate lungs. Their trust in me as a competent and loving caregiver is vital, and provides the parents with needed security and confidence. I've been told, "You are the only one I can leave the baby with."

If there are small children in the family, I may take them to the park or help facilitate play-dates with friends. I have picked kids up from preschool, taken them to the library for story hour, or done the shopping together, giving mom some quiet time at home. Discussing these needs prenatally can help the potential doula know whether she is comfortable performing the tasks the particular family will need postpartum. Family friends are wonderful in this role, as they are already known and trusted by both children and parents.

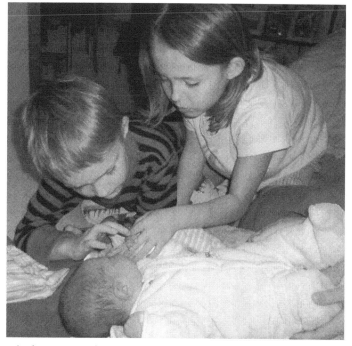

The beginning of a lifetime as part of a family —Photo credit: Jami Hornby

WHAT'S IMPORTANT TO THE MOTHER?

The bottom line is: what's important to the mother? How can I assist her to rest and let go, for these few short weeks, of many of her routine duties? She may be concerned about the dog's welfare, or the cleanliness of the rugs, or having her children's rooms kept tidy. The doula's work is to listen carefully to what she says and what she implies. Many women are uncomfortable asking for, or receiving, help from others, so we must become aware of the subtleties of communication. Sometimes a woman will say that she needs to do a particular chore, and I will quickly say, "Oh, I'll be happy to do that for you." It may take a little conditioning, but most women eventually begin to enjoy being served! You may remind her that this is a brief respite from normal reality, and she can relax and be the queen for the moment; it won't last forever.

If I'm asked to do a certain task, such as to make the beds in the children's rooms or water the garden, I will keep this in mind for future visits, and do it regularly. Once I recognize the areas needing consistent attention, I try to accommodate those needs routinely. In this way, our relationship grows as the parents realize my commitment and level of conscientious care. They come to trust my professionalism and integrity, and feel comfortable expressing their needs.

Chapter 14

FEEDING THE FAMILY

When I arrive at a postpartum home, I generally check in with the mom about how things are going. Among my first questions will be, "Have you had breakfast (lunch)?" or "Would you like a snack? A cup of tea or some more water?" Good nutrition and plenty of fluids are necessary for the mother's recovery and ongoing health and vitality. In some cases, I routinely prepare breakfast or lunch, or make salads to keep refrigerated for later. Family members don't always remember how hungry a nursing mother may become, and I have at times arrived to find that a woman hasn't eaten in hours. She really appreciates my attention to her personal needs, and my willingness to cook scrambled eggs or oatmeal, heat up leftovers, prepare sandwiches or colorful and healthy snacks, served in bed. One mom told me, "I can't remember the last time someone made lunch for me!"

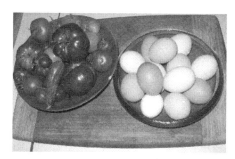

Fresh and simple foods support health for the whole family —Photo credit: Salle Webber

It can be difficult for a new mother to find the time to eat a full meal, but breastfeeding generates a healthy appetite. I encourage families to stock up on finger-foods and easy-to-eat snacks, such as fruits, vegetables, nuts, cheese sticks, whole-grain crackers or cereal bars. Mothers often become hungry during the night, and I recommend keeping a snack by the bed. A piece of fruit, a peanut butter sandwich, granola bar or something else that does not need refrigeration can help keep her energy up without requiring a trip to the kitchen (or waking an exhausted partner).

Seasonal fruits and vegetables are wonderful foods for women whose bodies are healing. I have frequently been asked to cut a melon into bite-sized pieces to keep in the refrigerator as a delicious and juicy snack. Grapes, apples, oranges, carrots, tomatoes, avocado, and so many other fruits and vegetables can be beautifully arranged on a plate with perhaps a few crackers, chunks of cheese, or a cookie. Emotionally sensitive postpartum women appreciate seeing beauty everywhere, and will notice it in the food you serve to them.

Remember that it is time-consuming to stand at the kitchen counter and wash and cut fruits and vegetables. New moms should stay off their feet when possible, yet they need the best nutrition. In some families, I do dinner preparation, such as readying vegetables for cooking, making salads, cooking a pot of rice, or putting a casserole into the oven. Once I was asked by exhausted parents to find something in the kitchen to cook for them. The cupboards were rather bare, but I put together a vegetable stew using what was there, both fresh and canned, and they pronounced it fabulously good! Another family asked several times a week for tuna-noodle casserole, their favorite "comfort food." Still another enjoyed having a chicken with potatoes and veggies put in the oven to roast before I left in the afternoon … an easy one-pot meal.

Clients often ask me what I like to cook, or what I'd suggest, so I have ideas of simple and nourishing options that I feel confident about. If they want something specific, I may ask how they like it prepared. I have a pretty good repertoire of vegetarian as well as meat dishes, and I love to serve fresh vegetables. Each doula should be clear about her cooking availability and/or limitations. Serious vegetarians may recoil at the sight of meat, and won't want to prepare it. Be clear about this with potential clients.

If there are small children in the family, they may have different food needs. Inquire of the parents what the children's eating routines are. Some eat whenever hungry. Some are allowed certain snacks between meals. Some have separate dinners from their parents, while others eat with mom and dad. I've known children who switched between grilled cheese sandwiches and macaroni and cheese … only. Sweet fruits, like berries and grapes, are popular finger foods, as are cheese sticks, crackers, or warm green peas. Sippy-cups of milk, diluted juice, or water help keep the child hydrated. Each family will have their own style of eating, and we work within the family's comfort zone. Keeping small children well fed with familiar foods is part of helping them to feel secure within their changing world.

Sometimes friends will offer to provide the new family with regular dinner deliveries after the birth, often known as a "meal tree." I recommend asking a trusted friend to be the coordinator, providing that friend's phone number or email address to all those interested in participating. Offer information about the family's food preferences and limitations. Remind those generous cooks that mom needs wholesome, simple, and

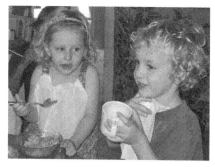

Keeping children's nutritional needs met helps them make the adjustment to the newborn's arrival —Photo credit: Aerielle Webber

nutritious foods. If there are foods that have proven irritating to mother or infant, ask friends to leave those ingredients out. Ask the coordinator to schedule deliveries, stretching it out for several weeks if possible, not necessarily every day, as leftovers will pile up (everyone's so generous!). I've found that friends appreciate knowing what the family really likes to eat, to avoid waste or disappointment. I encourage families to allow their community to assist them, to welcome these gifts of lovingly offered food. Everyone desires to help the new family, and this is a very functional and appreciated way to serve.

Chapter 15

INFANT CARE

The newborn human being is a large presence in a humble body. Though the impact of her arrival is monumental, her power immense, she is in a helpless and needy physical state. Less developed than other full-term mammals, she exerts voluntary control over her sucking muscles, but her limbs and most of her body are not under her conscious control. She is without fur and would surely become dangerously cold without clothing. As her organ systems are still maturing, she may experience digestive discomfort and, unlike some of her mammalian counterparts, need to be held, consoled, and burped.

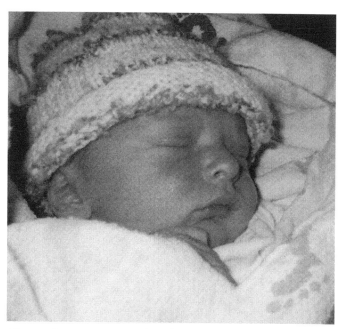

The newborn exists somewhere between heaven and earth—
Photo credit: Aerielle Webber

We are told that since humans have such large brains, they must be born before their heads are too big to get through the mother's birth canal. They are developmentally immature at birth, and for the first three months of life are learning to hold their heads up and roll over; not like a foal or calf that is walking on wobbly legs within minutes of birth, and can come and go from the nipple at will! The first three months after birth are truly the fourth trimester for a human mammal.

NEEDS OF THE NEWBORN

A newborn baby may do little other than sleep and feed. Often, she will appear peaceful, seem to digest easily, and fall asleep at the breast or in arms. The new mother will be able to rest and recuperate from the birth with a mellow baby next to her. We tend the little one gently, respecting her need for warmth and tenderness and low levels of stimulation. This period may last two weeks or more. Often at about two weeks, a new stage begins where the child appears to be more aware of her physical body, to suddenly feel everything, and to tell us about it! I have seen many parents surprised and concerned by this abrupt change. It seems the child becomes somehow more fully incarnated, more present in her body, and begins to experience the world as something different from whence she came.

On the other hand, some babies are born with eyes wide open, crying vigorously, very much awakened by the birth process. This child may appear hungry before the appearance of breast milk, not fully satisfied by the rich, but small-in-colostrum. She may be quite vocal and squirmy.

In any case, the primary needs of the infant are to be fed and kept warm; to urinate, eliminate meconium and then newborn stools;

to sleep, many hours a day; and experience human connection. A secure and calm environment allows the newborn to slowly open up to her surroundings.

FEEDING THE BABY

Many newborns breastfeed easily and naturally. Others have challenges, due to being born prematurely, the mother receiving drugs during birth, nipples that are flat or inverted, separation of child from mother, and other issues. Sometimes it just requires patience and practice. The doula can help by settling the nursing couple comfortably in a quiet place, providing water and pillows, and observing.

If the baby seems to be struggling, perhaps it's a positioning problem. Is the baby's head supported? Is she belly-to-belly with her mom? Is the baby being brought in close enough to latch on deeply? Maybe mom could gently knead her breast to express a bit of milk to touch the newborn lips, thus getting baby's attention. If we strive to recognize the baby's experience, we may be able to offer ideas that work. See the chapter "Breastfeeding Support" for more specific information.

Some babies are bottle fed, and this skill is generally easy to master. The infant needs to be held close and given good head and neck support. A pillow under the baby and under the arms of the adult can be helpful for good positioning and relaxed muscles. Elevate the baby's head to assist swallowing and digestion. Offer the bottle gently but persistently, and stop the feeding every ounce or so for an attempt at a burp. The flow of milk from the bottle is fast, and the infant may become uncomfortably full without short breaks. See "The Breastfed Baby's First Bottle" for more tips on bottle-feeding.

If the infant is premature with undeveloped sucking muscles and coordination, he will most likely be hospitalized until he reaches stability, being fed with a pediatric syringe or a finger-feeding tube. Parents are taught these feeding techniques by hospital personnel prior to going home.

It is important to know that breastfed babies need to nurse frequently, often every one and a half to three hours. A breastfed baby may also "cluster feed," cueing to nurse every 30 to 45 minutes for a few hours, before sleeping for 4 or 5. "Watch baby, not the clock" is a good rule to share with breastfeeding mothers, as a strict feeding schedule could lead to breastfeeding problems later on. Formula is slower to digest and may keep a newborn's hunger at bay for three to four hours.

In the early days of life, an exceptionally sleepy baby may need to be awakened for feeding, though it is sometimes difficult to get a sleepy baby latched on to the breast. Generally I'm not inclined to wake a sleeping baby, but if there is any concern about weight gain, jaundice, or failure to thrive adequately, I certainly support parents in encouraging the baby to eat frequently. Babies who are skin-to-skin with mother will usually rouse on their own, but others may need to be stimulated

Some ways of waking a newborn to nurse or bottle-feed are unwrapping and undressing him, changing the diaper, touching and talking, stroking his limbs, as well as stroking the cheeks to stimulate the sucking reflex. After compressing or massaging the breast to begin the flow, a few drops of milk expressed onto his lips may also stir his interest. While at the breast, a gentle squeeze of the breast keeps milk flowing and can keep a sleepy baby eating. It is not uncommon in the first few days of a child's life that he needs to be reminded to eat, guided to the breast and onto the nipple, or given a bottle.

BURPING THE BABY

It is important to a newborn's comfort to move any gas bubbles through and out of his body. There are several good burping positions: holding the baby against the shoulder, and patting or rubbing the back; sitting the baby up in your lap, with good chin support, patting or rubbing gently. Try stroking the back upward from hips to shoulders. I like to hold babies upright against my chest and gently but firmly pat their backs, and often the gas comes out in this position. It can be a matter of movement: just shifting position can often allow the burp to be released. It's wise to try burping once or twice during the feeding, as well as after. Often if a baby doesn't burp but falls asleep, he will be awakened a while later by the need to burp. Some breastfed babies burp infrequently, since with a good latch, little air is taken in, and the milk is easily assimilated. With observation, each mother will recognize her particular child's tendencies.

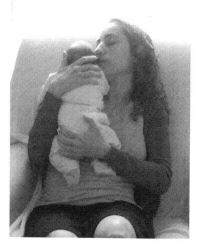

Mom and baby both enjoy relaxed feedings with plenty of burp and snuggle breaks —Photo credit: Salle Webber

Gas also exits the baby's body via the anus. Farting frequently relieves a squirming infant. If he's disturbed by uncomfortable bubbles moving through his intestinal tract, he won't be able to nurse or bottle-feed with the necessary focus. Everyone cheers when a newborn farts!

HOW TO HELP

As the doula or caregiver, you can offer to burp the baby during a break in the feeding, or change the diaper if needed. If baby gets too sleepy, a diaper change can be a good way of stimulating her to continue the feeding. Also, should the mother and child have difficulty getting latched on, and one or both become upset, you may offer to hold and soothe the baby while mom regroups, then try again when everyone's calmed down. The doula's ability to calm the infant is vital. The newborn may wish to suck on a pacifier or a clean finger, or her own fist, to bring order to her inner disorder. Sucking brings a feeling of rhythm rather than chaos into the body, and can relieve digestive discord. Parents often have concerns about using pacifiers. Generally with moderate and purposeful use, they can be soothing and calming for the infant. However, please note that the American Academy of Pediatrics recommends delaying pacifier use until a breastfed infant is four weeks of age so that it will not interfere with the establishment of breastfeeding.

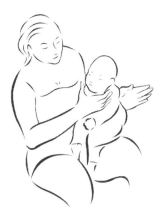

Sometimes we use an upright position to help a baby burp, with good chin and head support —Illustration credit: Ken Tackett

Patience is a key factor in early nursing. Many women have given up on breastfeeding for lack of an informed and encouraging support person. You, the doula or friendly helper, can make the difference in the breastfeeding pair's experience by maintaining a positive, helpful, and persevering attitude and presence. Please read thoroughly the chapter "Breastfeeding Support." Professionals can find other ways of educating themselves, such as Nursing Mothers Counsel, La Leche League, Breastfeeding USA, or Australian Breastfeeding Association groups, lectures by lactation consultants, or by reading some of the excellent books available on the subject. Breastfeeding support is one of the most important functions of the postpartum doula.

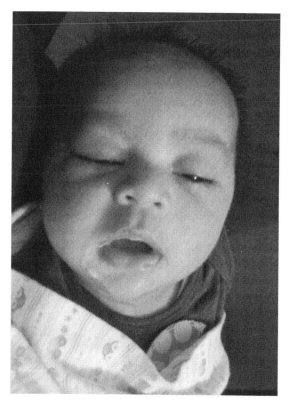

Ahhh…full of mommy's milk —Photo credit: Nisa Sampior

SPITTING UP

Babies might spit up small amounts of milk, due to gas, over-feeding, receiving too fast a flow, gulping, or just because. It is not a problem unless it is consistently projectile, abundant, and upsets the child, appearing painful. This can be a sign of reflux, digestive difficulty, or illness. The healthcare provider should be contacted if it is worrisome. Spitting up seems to relieve some pressure or just comes up with a burp. It's perfectly OK, and it's wise to wear an old cloth diaper over your shoulder, especially around those babies who seem to spit up often. They will need their mouths and chins wiped afterward, as well. Serious and excessive throwing up is addressed in the chapter called "Colic, Reflux, and Thrush."

MODERN DIAPERING

You came the morning after Sara and I got home from the hospital. The evening before I'd tried to put my cloth diaper on my little premature baby and it totally engulfed her, so in tears I turned to the disposable diapers the hospital had given me. I remember feeling so relieved that you would be there the next day to solve the cloth-diaper dilemma, and, as you did with all problems, you quietly, calmly, lovingly showed me how to fold the diaper without covering Sara's tummy button.

—Evie, first-time mom

Diapering is easier than ever and generally there are several kinds of diapers to choose from: disposable, with a choice of regular, or "natural" — bleach- and gel-free; cloth diapers washed and dried at home; cloth diapers from a diaper service; or the latest option, compostable disposables. Cloth diapers require a diaper cover, of which there are many great styles, generally with Velcro closures. These must be laundered at home, and several pairs in each size are necessary. Cloth diapering is a wonderful option, and the diaper services are generally very good, delivering spanking clean diapers to the door and taking away the dirty ones, with no rinsing on your part. Compostables seem to be a responsible choice, also available and composted by some of the diaper services. Disposable diapers can be found in many styles, sizes, and brands, and are especially useful for traveling or day-care situations.

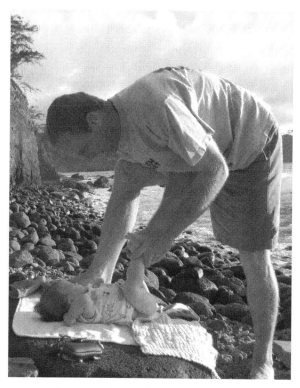

Diaper change at the beach —Photo credit: Erin Baldwin Brown

Each family will make its own choice, and the doula's job is to support that. If, however, a disposable-wrapped newborn is experiencing rashes, one could suggest trying a cloth diaper for a while, or switching to the "natural" disposable diaper. Many of the disposable wipes on the market contain alcohol, which tends to reduce the moisture in newborn skin. I suggest using alcohol-free wipes or warm water on a washcloth. One helpful idea for those who want to use water to clean the baby during diaper changes, but don't have a sink close to the changing area: get a thermos, fill with hot water each morning, and provide a small bowl and a pile of baby washcloths. Water can be poured into the bowl for each change, and dumped out when you have a free hand. Such simple suggestions can be a big help to new parents. It's a fortunate baby who is cleaned with warm water and wears cloth diapers, but it's no longer the norm. Go with the flow.

If you're not practiced with today's diapers, it is necessary to get some experience. Our local diaper service has a newborn size diaper that can be easily folded lengthwise in thirds. Put it inside the diaper cover, and fold extra length under, away from baby's body, in the front for boys, in the back for girls. Wrap up with diaper cover and Velcro closed. *Voilà!* Easy! There are other ways to position the diaper as well. You can find what you prefer, and see what the new mom likes. Just be sure that the cover is enclosing the cloth around the legs—no cloth sticking out to allow leakage. In the same way, the disposable diaper must be opened up fully around tiny baby legs. There is usually gathering around the legs to hold the diaper snug there, where leakage often occurs. Fasten loosely around the baby's waist, and until the umbilicus falls off, try to put the diaper beneath the navel to avoid irritation. Be willing and ready to change the baby's clothes whenever necessary, because diapers may leak no matter how good you are at diapering!

BOWEL MOVEMENTS AND CONSTIPATION

The first bowel movements consist of meconium, a tarry, black substance that lines the intestines of the baby in the womb. After several days, the consistency and color will begin to change to the seedy, loose, yellow or brownish stools that will continue with breast-feeding until solid foods are introduced. A breastfed infant may also have green stools. If the infant is exhibiting fussiness as well, this could be a sign of digestive issues but otherwise may be within the range of normal.

Infants don't typically get seriously hungry until their intestines are cleared of the meconium, which beautifully coincides with the beginning of the copious flow of mother's milk, around the third day or so.

Meconium is sticky and messy. Launder carefully. My husband discovered that a cold water and salt soak helped get out the stains. Especially in the first few days, a new mother needs to have these things taken care of for her.

Newborns who receive formula instead of (or to supplement) breast milk may have bowel movements that are thicker, pasty or formed, and generally greenish or brownish in color. Sometimes constipation, or hard and dry stools, occurs with formula feeding. If this appears to be the case, the parents must reevaluate their choice of formula, perhaps changing from cow's milk-based to soy-based, or choosing a no-iron or hypoallergenic formula, or one of the organic varieties. They should consult their baby's doctor.

If a breastfeeding newborn is not producing stools in the first weeks of life, it may be a sign of poor nursing, and requires attention. Around six weeks of age we often see a change to fewer stools.

This is normal. But should an infant go several days without a bowel movement, he can become very uncomfortable. On the other hand, he may be fine. The bottom line is how is baby behaving? Does he appear unusually uncomfortable, kicking his legs and arching, with a hard belly? Squirming and can't settle down? If a few days have gone by without a poop, this can be the cause. Lay him on his changing table, and slowly and rhythmically raise his legs and hips off the table, and lower again. This can stimulate the intestines into action. Leg rotations also are helpful, circling the hips gently. Or you can bend and straighten the baby's knees, in bicycle fashion. Massaging along the outside of the thigh also stimulates the large intestine. Removing the diaper while doing these exercises, allowing air to touch the skin, as well as providing freedom of movement, can help to encourage a bowel movement. A rectal thermometer inserted gently, according to directions, can often provide the necessary stimulation to the system.

I remember one adopted baby girl who was receiving formula. She didn't poop for several days and the parents were worried. We took off her diaper and let her kick freely on her changing table. We moved her legs around and gently massaged her belly and thighs. After a while, sure enough, she pooped! The next day, we tried it again, and were again rewarded after about twenty minutes. This became a morning ritual, and she routinely waited for this naked and relaxing time to empty her bowels.

Another way that a breastfeeding mother can help an infant who seems to have sluggish bowels is through her own diet. I often encourage moms to drink some prune juice, a couple of glasses each day, or eat dried apricots or other dried fruits. Generally within 36 hours of this, the baby will be relieved. It's not uncommon, when I ask a mom with a mildly constipated baby, if she herself is at all constipated, for her to answer, "Yes!" Remember that in many ways, the mother and child are still one. Encouraging mothers to improve their diets by eating smaller amounts of processed foods and more fruits, vegetables, and whole grains will support the health and long-term well-being of both mothers and babies.

Breastfed babies will often, though not always, have six or eight or more bowel movements a day, perhaps in almost every diaper. This can change abruptly, to once or twice a day, after a few weeks. This is normal. It's also not unusual for a newborn to establish a once-a-day-or-less schedule of elimination. The important thing is to observe the baby for signs of comfort/discomfort, to be sure there are lots of wet diapers, and the baby is continuing to gain well. Generally, constipation is a problem of formula-fed babies, and infrequently seen in exclusively breastfed infants. The baby receiving a diet of infant formula is more likely to have one or two bowel movements per day, and should have at least six to eight wet diapers a day

DRESSING THE NEWBORN

Newborns need warmth. Their bodies are thin, they frequently have very little hair to warm their heads, and they aren't physically active enough to generate heat. It is currently popular to say, "Dress the baby as you dress yourself." This may encourage parents to under-dress their little ones. I routinely see newborns wearing only one layer of light clothing, with one thin receiving blanket over them when they nap. Ideally, a newborn will wear a "onesie" or t-shirt, with a nightgown or full-body suit, as well as socks and a hat, and be wrapped in a light blanket. In cool weather, or an air-conditioned home, an additional layer is appropriate. Hats are important, as body heat is lost through the head.

A simple way to explain this is in terms of calories. The newborn receives a specific amount of calories from his milk. Ideally, these

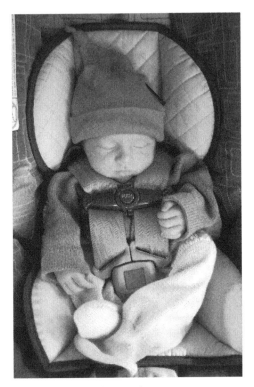

Dressed and ready to ride —Photo credit: Daniella Sandler

calories are used for physical growth and development. However, if a child's body is cold, his internal thermostat will activate to warm his body. This requires calories. Clearly, then, those calories are not available for growth. I have seen, again and again, that mothers who dress their babies very warmly, with sweaters and hats and cozy blankets, see rapid growth and weight-gain in their infants. Those babies who are particularly lightly dressed seem fine but do not gain weight rapidly.

Overheating can be a concern as well. Cotton blankets are preferable to fleecy synthetics, allowing more breathability and airflow. The home should not be exceptionally warm, but perhaps slightly above normal in cold climates. Primarily, the child should be dressed well to accommodate her particular stage of life. Feel her neck, torso, hands and feet for clues about her temperature. If hot and clammy, remove a layer of clothes or blankets. If cool, add a layer. A baby kept skin-to-skin in bed with her mother may only need a light blanket on top. Very often, I will ask where the baby's hats are kept, and I'll pop one on her head. I may put another light, non-fluffy blanket over a sleeping baby, modeling this concept for the parents. I make it a point to bundle up babies in my care. It may generate discussion on the topic of dressing, a very good thing to talk about.

On a cool autumn day I began assisting a young mother with a four-week-old son. I arrived to find the baby napping in a bassinet, wearing a onesie with a light receiving blanket over him. I suggested dressing him more warmly, including a hat, as I explained to the mom that her baby needed to use his calories to grow, rather than to keep himself warm. As there were concerns about weight-gain and milk production, my explanation made sense to her and she agreed to my suggestion. Her mother-in-law had stayed with them for the first four weeks, shopping, cooking, cleaning, doing laundry, keeping the household running comfortably as the young parents adjusted. She had suggested several times that the infant could be dressed more warmly, but the parents didn't listen. They loved her and respected the fact that she had

*raised five children, but it took the word of a paid professional
to get their attention. Certainly the grandma's ability to refrain
from telling the young parents how to do their job made her
a welcomed helper. But they did not fully utilize her wisdom.
They began dressing the baby more warmly, and his growth level
increased soon after.*

SKIN CARE

The doula should know about newborn skin care. Rashes may
come and go on any part of the body, and generally are not a problem. Newborn skin is especially permeable, so it is wise to read labels
on soaps and lotions, and avoid products with long lists of chemical
ingredients. The skin is sensitive and affected by temperature, clothing, dirty diapers, or drooled milk. Unless there are pus-filled pimples,
there is not typically a need for concern. Many skin rashes go away
in a few hours, or after a bath or warm face-wipe.

The diaper area, however, requires vigilance because of the skin's
contact with urine and feces, sometimes for hours at a time. This
area needs to be well cleaned with each diaper change, to maintain
the health of the delicate skin. This is true even if there is no visible
matter on the baby's bottom; wash him anyway. Should diaper rash
occur, and it is not uncommon, there are many products available
to help: lotions, ointments, or simple cornstarch. Early treatment of
diaper rash is best, as it can become persistent and painful. With
each change, thoroughly dry the skin before putting on the clean
diaper. Allowing the diaper area to air out for a while before putting
on a fresh diaper is not only beneficial to the skin, but pleasurable

for baby as well.

Sometimes diaper rash can signal the presence of thrush, a yeasty condition discussed more fully in the chapter "Colic, Reflux, and Thrush." This rash tends to be spotty, rather than spread across the skin, and accompanied by white spots in the mouth. The mother's nipples will be sore and not improving normally. If this seems to be a possibility, encourage the mother to have the doctor check for thrush, and treat if necessary.

Around three to four weeks, "newborn acne" will appear. This consists of pimples on the face, and sometimes on the chest and torso as well. Some babies have just a few pimples, and others have many. They can appear overnight, and though this is mentioned in the paperwork sent home by the hospital, many parents are taken by surprise. They can be reassured that this is normal and will disappear within a few weeks. This rash is the result of the elimination of hormones the baby received from the mother in the womb. No special care is necessary, beyond gently wiping the face with a warm washcloth a couple of times a day to calm the redness.

Some parents enjoy massaging their infant, with olive, almond, or another high-quality oil. This can be done after a bath, and brings the child into a beautifully relaxed state. Books are available with specific techniques, or simple gentle kneading and stroking is fine. This is a wonderful way to connect more deeply with your baby's physical being, feel her muscles, where she may hold tension, where she feels robust, where she is sensitive. You may gaze into each other's eyes and see the universe unfold.

CARE OF THE UMBILICUS

The umbilical stump frequently drops off between one and two weeks, though it may take longer. There are various ideas about its care. Commonly, mothers are advised to clean the area once or twice a day with alcohol. This is easily done with a Q-tip, and the stump can be gently lifted to allow the alcohol onto the gooey tissue, helping it to dry out. Dabbing around the outside, on healthy skin, does not help. Sometimes new parents are squeamish about this, and the doula can demonstrate by exposing the rotting flesh and applying alcohol as a drying agent.

Some hospitals apply an indigo-colored disinfectant to the area, and advise parents that they need do nothing more. Some care providers suggest leaving it alone entirely. It may take longer to drop off without help, but generally it's fine either way, whatever the parents are most comfortable with. It will have a mild fleshy smell, but requires medical attention if the site becomes really foul-smelling or exudes pus. Be aware of keeping the diaper below the umbilicus to avoid uncomfortable rubbing.

BATHING THE BABY

Before the cord stump drops off, we want to keep the umbilical area dry to avoid the possibility of bacteria entering the open wound. For this reason, we do not immerse the child in water until it is healed. It is only necessary to clean the diaper area well with each diaper change, and wipe the face and hands occasionally with a damp washcloth. If the mother desires a more thorough sponge bath, be aware of not letting the baby become chilled. Try undressing one part of the body at a time, wash and dry the area, and cover with a towel before moving on to the next part. If the umbilical area should get wet from a diaper or in bathing, a hair dryer set on low can be helpful to dry it out and speed healing. Be aware that there are different beliefs and cultural customs surrounding bathing, so be flexible if the parents are quite clear about what they want to do.

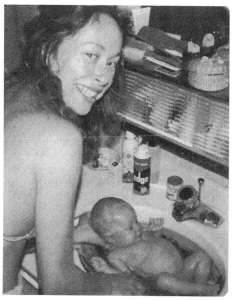

Babies don't require extra equipment; a bathroom sink can easily be a baby tub—
Photo credit: Leo Webber

The time for the first bath has come once the cord stump area has fully dried, with no further risk of infection. I believe that the initial bath experience should be geared toward pleasure rather than focused on washing. Ideally, the child will come to love her bath, and it will become a place for relaxation and comfort. Timing is essential. Bathe the baby when she is awake and alert, but not hungry. After a feeding is good, before she gets sleepy.

Warm the room if the weather is cool. Plastic infant tubs are useful, but creative parents may also use the sink. Fill with comfortably warm water, and then gently lower the naked baby in, feet first, allowing adjustment time. Keep one hand under her upper back and neck at all times. Spoon water over her exposed parts with your hand or washcloth, keeping her warm all over. Speak in soft happy tones, and move in a relaxed fashion, giving her confidence in her security here in this element. Use a thin washcloth or just your hands. Her face can be gently washed with plain water. Gently wash her body, especially in the creases of her elbows, armpits, under her neck, backs of knees, thighs, between fingers and toes. Lift her carefully forward to wash her back. The diaper area is really nourished by soaking and thorough washing. A drop of baby shampoo is enough to wash her hair, and then use the washcloth to rinse well. Do all this only as long as she is having fun. If it becomes too much, don't insist. She's not really dirty anyway.

Lift her out of the tub and directly into a cozy towel, perhaps the kind with built-in hood. You may have warmed the towel by putting it in the dryer for a few minutes beforehand. Dry and dress her without letting her get chilled. She may want to nurse for a few minutes after her bath, and will then most likely sleep well. A couple of baths a week are usually enough initially. I have given many babies their first baths, to help the new mother see how easy it is. It's fun and pleasant for baby, too, and she will smell so clean afterward.

THE NEED FOR SLEEP

Salle arrived a day or so after baby's birth and immediately
took my loudly crying newborn and soothed him to sleep. I still

have vivid memories of her gentle bounce. In awe, I would watch her soothe this new screaming infant into tranquility. I used to ask my husband, "how does she do that?" and then watch her carefully, hoping I could imitate her feet and the sway of her body as she lulled him to sleep. I always said that Salle could put a baby to sleep in a hurricane.

—Julie, first-time mom

Newborns require up to twenty hours of sleep daily. Some sleep more easily than others. My friend Ellen, after the birth of her first daughter, said, "Everyone told me they sleep twenty hours a day … but no one told me it would be in fifteen minute increments!" This was true of little Tara, though certainly not of all babies. In arms, or attached to a baby bundler or sling, Tara would sleep for hours! She simply could not tolerate being separated, and would awaken and cry within five minutes if put down. I used to vacuum the whole house with her attached to me, fast asleep. I believe if a baby needs to be held, hold her! She needs to develop a sense of security, of safety in the world, and will detach when ready. Children let us know when they're ready to move on to the next step in independent development. It's helpful to maintain an attitude of respecting the child's process, rather than insisting that she conform to our routines right away. For a newborn, the peaceful and relaxing experience of being soothed by the mother lays the foundation for the ability to self-soothe later on.

In general, babies do sleep longer and deeper, and remain more content, when we "wear" or hold them. The concept of Attachment Parenting includes this idea of constant physical contact. There are many varieties of baby carriers available commercially. My favorite is the Baby Bundler, a long piece of cotton fabric that is wrapped a certain way to attach the newborn to the caregiver's chest. It is extremely comfortable for both, and allows the caregiver to accomplish other tasks or to rest comfortably with a secure baby. Slings and other types of carriers are also available. They reduce stimulation and help newborns to sleep deeply. I particularly recommend bundlers to parents of fussy or high-need infants. The doula can care for the home at the same time as she cares for the infant when she wears him in a bundler. I have several, and share them with my clients, who frequently purchase their own.

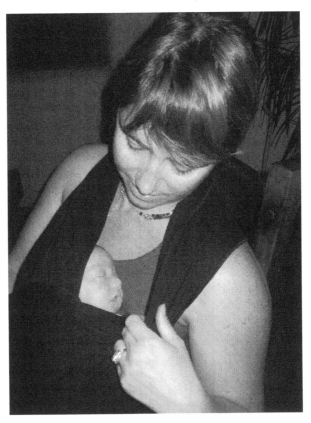

Wearing the baby allows both mother and infant to comfortably enjoy close physical contact —Photo credit: Bradley Brown

In our modern lives, women may spend many hours each day without anyone to help with household duties and infant care. When the doula holds the baby, mom has some time with arms free. When we handle some of the household chores, mom can relax and give her child lots of attention, or settle in for a nap with baby. We encourage mom to sleep when baby sleeps, because she will most likely be awake when baby is awake!

Once the baby is deeply asleep, we may lay him in his bassinet, cradle, basket, crib, infant seat, or whatever is available. Put him down gently, in a warm sleeper; he no longer has the warmth of your body close to him. Currently doctors are recommending babies be put on their backs to sleep, though for decades the recommended sleeping position was on the belly. It is believed that Sudden Infant Death Syndrome is more prevalent with stomach sleeping and that babies may suffocate in their bedding and blankets. Unfortunately, many babies are uncomfortable on their backs, and startle themselves awake frequently. As a result, they may have a more difficult time staying asleep and need an adult nearby to help them settle. Some babies, especially those with reflux, are more comfortable sleeping on a wedge with their heads elevated.

Frequently, a well-fed and burped baby will nap for up to two hours in her own bed, but it can be unpredictable. The need to burp can cause bodily sensations that disturb the child enough to wake her. If we have her in a bundler, we can pat her back and bounce a bit, enough to get out the burp and lull her back into a deep sleep. As we get to know each newborn individually, we will understand what each one needs in order to get deep rest. Often I spend several hours a day holding a sleeping infant. This is an excellent use of my time. I have been told that the baby is like soft butter after a nap in my arms!

It's important to understand that infants need to sleep and eat regularly, around the clock. The idea that she has her "days and nights mixed up," as parents sometimes say, is inaccurate. Her body requires cycles of sleeping and eating, in one and a half to three hour intervals, with short periods of being awake. Occasionally an infant will sleep for four hours at a stretch, and for this a mother rejoices. But we must be respectful of baby's personal rhythm. She doesn't wake up at three a.m. to annoy us, but because her body needs fuel.

It seems that newborns sometimes prefer being awake at night, when stimulation is low: the phone isn't ringing, TV and lights are off, and outside noises are lessened. The child has her mother's full attention. It is a safe and comfortable space to begin exploring her world. This is a precious time for mother and child to learn more about each other and to connect intimately. Remind her to enjoy it; these weeks will soon be over.

"A WELL-RESTED BABY RESTS WELL"

In many homes where I work, after perhaps two or three weeks of parenthood, it's usually the father who announces one day, "We're going to keep the baby awake during the day so he'll sleep better at night. He's sleeping so much during the day, he's not tired enough at night." The plan is to stimulate the child when he begins to get sleepy in daytime, keeping him up. This is a perfect example of adult logic. Unfortunately, babies are pre-logical and this theory is doomed for failure. We end up with a cranky, over-stimulated child whose need to sleep is thwarted. He will be unable to sleep well at night because his rhythm is off. I patiently explain this when I hear the theory, but sometimes they must try it anyway. Often the mother more quickly understands what the baby is trying to teach because of her intimacy with him.

> *Years ago, I was helping Jenny and Larry, both about 40, with their first child, Chelsea. When she was four weeks old, I arrived one Monday morning. "What a great day we had yesterday," they told me. "We went sailing on a yacht with 20 people; it was sunny, windy, clear and beautiful. The baby slept all afternoon, being held by all our friends. She was great!" I answered that I was happy for them, and wondered how the evening at home went, after the sail. "Oh!," they exclaimed, "Chelsea cried for hours, very difficult. We didn't know what was wrong." I wasn't surprised to hear this. When a baby is over-stimulated, or in a situation that's too much for her to handle, her normal response is to shut down and go to sleep. It's self-protection. Later, in the security of home, this tiny girl needed to release all the tension she absorbed in the sun and wind and crowd of unfamiliar people. She was inconsolable until she let it all out, then she could rest.*

I see variations on this theme regularly. Let me add, too, that some babies, like some adults, are far more sensitive than others. It's just how they are. A particular newborn may require quiet in his sleeping area, be unable to be away from mom for long, need to nap against her (or dad's or doula's) chest, or be upset by going into stores or in the car. My recommendation is to go with the child's temperament, let him be who he is, especially during those precious first six weeks, when mother and child are recovering from birth and adjusting to life. Keep in mind what a tremendous transition this little person has made, and respect his need to follow the demands of his body.

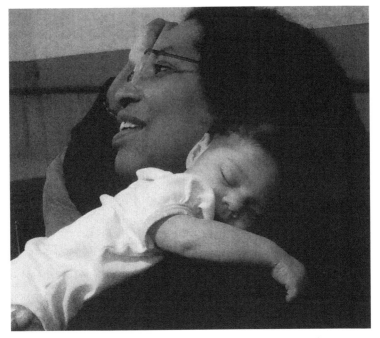

Newborns fit into the ongoing life of the extended family, sleeping easily in relaxed and caring arms —Photo credit: Buddy Rizzio

SLEEPING ISSUES

There is endless controversy about where the baby should sleep. It appears to me that it can be distressing to a newborn to be too far from his mother. The mother herself is psychically connected to the child and very tuned in to him. In short, they need one another, physically and emotionally. They had been sharing a body up to the moment of birth. It is in the child's best interest that the mother is close by, listening, observing, and responding to the infant, as she knows him best.

Many parents are comfortable and happy sharing their bed with their newborn. It is easy to respond to the child's sounds and movements, and to sit up in bed or nurse lying down. Mom doesn't have to get up and go to another room to fetch a crying baby. She can tend to him before he awakens to the point of crying, and both of them remain calm and sleepy. This is how we have done it for thousands of years. After all, if the baby was left alone in the next cave, he might not have survived the night! For comfort, warmth, security, and safety, we have kept our families close together at night throughout human history (McKenna & McDade, 2005).

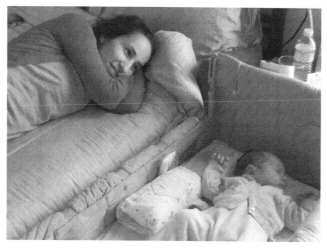

The co-sleeper provides parents easy access to their babies
—Photo credit: Salle Webber

For parents who want the baby close, but are uncomfortable sharing their bed, a co-sleeper is a good alternative. It is a baby-sized bed which attaches to the parents' bed, giving the infant his own space while providing easy access to mother. A cradle, bassinet, or crib next to mom's side of the bed, or somewhere in the room, can become baby's sleeping area, and his sounds can be heard and evaluated. Babies can be noisy sleepers, and it can take time to understand which grunts and cries indicate need for attention. Some parents have spoken of the tendency to awaken to baby's every movement, until they gradually became able to recognize differences in the baby's sounds, and not respond to every whimper. Accumulated sleep deprivation assists the parents in developing this skill of discernment, and after a while they awaken only when necessary.

> *I helped Lynnette after her third child was born. She had figured out with the first two that she needed a certain distance between herself and baby, or she wouldn't sleep soundly. She put Joshua's cradle in the bathroom hallway, as that gave her just the amount of space from him that she needed. She still had easy access to him and could hear his call. This is what worked for her.*

Every family has its own style and philosophy. Some parents want the newborn in his own room, and will use a baby monitor. I personally prefer that a newborn be close to others when sleeping, but I do support each family in making choices appropriate to themselves. However, if they wish to discuss it, I will share my thoughts that babies need continual human contact. Observing newborns, we notice that their breathing is irregular, and long pauses may occur between breaths. One theory says that infants are re-stimulated into the next breath by the sensory awareness of the presence of another person. They may smell, hear, feel, or sense that presence, and it allows them to continue breathing and, hence, living, as the newborn cannot survive alone. Baby monitors allow us to hear the baby, but the baby can't hear us, and they don't tell us when a child is not breathing. I prefer to keep a sleeping infant near me, and I make it a practice to check regularly on a baby who is in my care if I'm in a different room.

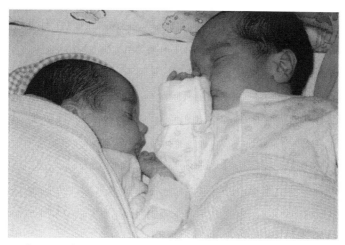

Sleeping close is especially comforting to twins, and all newborns need others close by —Photo credit: Fatima Kazimi

Ultimately, it may be a combination of sleeping styles that the family adopts. The baby may start out in her own bed, but after the first feeding, end up next to mom. Or there may be an extra bedroom, in which mom and baby make their nest for a few weeks, allowing dad to get a full night's sleep before facing the world each morning. It is a personal decision of the couple, and the doula's work is to support and honor their choices, as well as to offer suggestions when appropriate. Remember that this is the first time that new parents are facing these issues, so in many cases they are open to hearing how other families have worked things out. Keep it light and laugh as much as possible.

There are many stories of babies in distant orphanages who lie in cribs all day, with minimal human touch. Some of these children do not survive, though their bodies are sound. The human being is not designed to live alone. We are interdependent. Infants need constant care, as they are helpless. Receiving quick and loving responses gives a child the sense that the world is benevolent ... what a lovely way to approach life!

THE INFANT'S BIRTH EXPERIENCE

There are many procedures done routinely during hospital births that affect the infant. Anything that is done to the mother may act upon the newborn. An epidural, for example, is an injection of a local analgesic. While it decreases the mother's experience of contractions, it also may numb the mouth of the infant, similar to Novocain, making early feeding difficult or impossible.

Immediately after birth, there are often things done to the baby that preclude allowing him to rest on his mother's belly, and find his way to her breast. This ritual is frequently interrupted with medical procedures, cleaning, weighing, eye drops, sometimes isolation and observation, oxygen, x-rays, injections, and whatever else is deemed prudent. The bonding period is postponed, and both mother and child experience separation.

Some babies require extreme medical intervention, and this can wrench the heart of a parent, who longs to hold and comfort the child, but instead must wait helplessly as doctors do what they can to remedy a physical defect or save a tiny preemie.

No one can say for sure what a newborn feels, thinks, or senses, but I propose the possibility that some emotional trauma can occur for the infant in these cases. We know that the biological expectation of the newborn is to continue the close physical bond with its mother. Perhaps fear or a sense of insecurity or abandonment can result from the severing of this connection, compounded by the presence of strangers, new smells and unrecognized voices, and painful medical procedures.

What can we do for a child thus affected? Joseph Chilton Pearce, author, lecturer, and teacher, assures us that healing of birth trauma is possible, simply through loving attention and reassurance. Basically, the baby needs to be held a lot, and all her needs should be met kindly and quickly. If she cries inconsolably, try to console her anyway; let her know that you are there with her. Even though you can't always take away her pain, you will support her as she goes through what life offers.

The doula can provide hours of quiet baby holding. As we are skilled in the handling of newborns, we know how to help them become calm and surrender to sleep. Many newborns, especially those who have undergone birth trauma, desire to sleep in arms for several weeks, and will wake and fuss soon after being put down. My philosophy is to follow the baby's lead. If this is what she needs to be able to fully relax and go to sleep, then I am willing to give it. I have no expectations about when a baby should be ready to sleep on her own … I feel the baby will let us know when she's feeling secure enough to be alone.

THE DOULA'S PRESENCE

A calm, confident, quiet, and efficient presence is appropriate for the doula. We remain relaxed even when the baby is crying; even when the mother is crying, we exude a sense that all is well. We understand and honor what they're going through, and we know that it will pass, that to release is good and natural. We take the baby into our arms and soothe her with our soft touch and gentle rhythm. We swaddle her in our warmth, and allow her to fully relax and return to peacefulness. It eases the tension in a room immediately when a crying baby quiets. This is a tremendous gift you can offer, the ability to quickly and reliably soothe an infant. It seems that the newborns I care for sense the presence of all those before them that have rested against my chest, and they are calmed when I hold them.

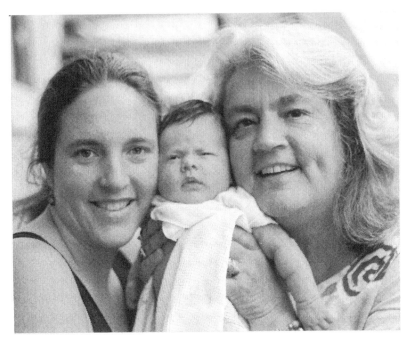

Three generations of females, the circle of life —Photo credit: Ed Sale

When dressing and diapering, I remain gentle and respectful, keeping baby as warm as possible, and maintaining a soft touch and comforting voice. No sense of urgency, though I am practiced and efficient. I try to model for the parents a genuine enjoyment of the work of baby care, a feeling of awe and appreciation as we witness this new life unfolding.

Chapter 16

BREASTFEEDING SUPPORT

Breastfeeding is as ancient as birth itself. It is the natural progression of gestation and delivery. Female bodies are programmed for this; we wouldn't have survived as a species without a built-in mechanism for infant nutrition. I dare say that our earliest foremothers never had the thought that maybe they "couldn't" breastfeed. They simply did what came naturally.

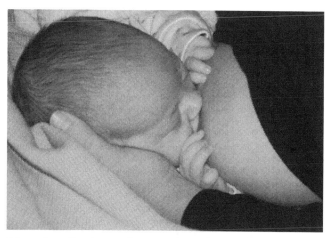

Home base for the newborn, a place of nourishment, warmth, and security —Photo credit: Joe Stearns

With the complexities of modern life has come a loss of trust in the body's innate capacities, and some women today feel anxious about their ability to succeed at breastfeeding. We have been shown images of smiling mothers holding bottles of formula in their chubby children's mouths, and we have been told the lie that this is the superior food for our infants. Nursing has been hidden for many decades, resulting in a lack of comfortable familiarity with the sight of a baby latched on to his mother's breast. We are now relearning what is ancient, and finding challenges along the way. The work of lactation support requires understanding of some of the more common barriers to nursing.

Frequently, questions about breastfeeding arrive right along with the baby. Many women have the expectation of nourishing their child naturally, but it remains a mystery until it actually is happening. There are a number of variables, making each nursing pair unique. The nature of the birth and recovery for both mother and infant are factors in early nursing and bonding. The shape and size of the mother's nipples (not breasts, nipples) can affect baby's latch and mother's comfort. The vigor of the infant affects the amount of stimulation the breasts receive, prompting the let-down of the first fluid provided to the newborn, the protective and protein-rich colostrum, and promoting continuing milk production. The level of encouragement for breastfeeding from those around the mother is a crucial factor, as well as the health of the mother, diet, age, attitude and expectation; all are part of the whole picture.

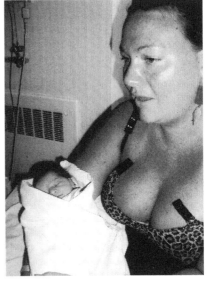

When the milk comes in, the breast may seem bigger than the baby's head
—Photo credit: Aerielle Webber

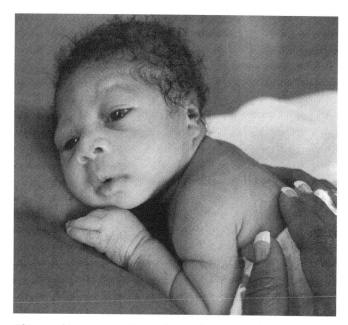

Skin-to-skin contact allows the newborn to find her way to the nipple when she's ready —Photo credit: Maggie Muir

Ideally, an infant is put to the breast within the first hour after birth, taking advantage of the physiological responses that are programmed into our mammalian bodies. Sucking comes naturally, and is rewarded with rich, thick colostrum, providing antibodies and proteins. The connection of mother and child outside the womb is established naturally, fluidly; it is the continuation of the relationship their bodies already know so well. Around the third day, after the colostrum has been fully received, and the breasts have been stimulated by lots of sucking, the flow of milk begins. Sometimes the milk comes in gently, sometimes like a burst dam, causing excessive and uncomfortable fullness. In any case, the baby's sweet mouth is eagerly ready, and lots of nursing is the correct response. Successful breastfeeding is established, and the mother's body gradually adjusts its milk production to the baby's intake.

That is the ideal situation, but in reality, there are many variables that can affect early breastfeeding. Some common experiences that may interfere with a smooth transition into nursing are medical interventions that result in separation of mother and child (such as when an infant needs supplemental oxygen); sedation of mother so she is unable to handle her baby right away (such as after a c-section); or use of an epidural during labor, which may interfere with sucking. Some babies are simply sleepy after the long journey of birth and show no urge to suck immediately. Premature infants may not have the muscular coordination to suck successfully, and are often fed with a bottle, cup, or finger-feeding tube for weeks. All these things can disrupt the establishment of successful nursing. Often support around the breastfeeding woman to keep trying long enough to establish the nursing relationship does not exist. But with persistence, in most cases, breastfeeding is absolutely possible. As doulas, we can provide the support that makes the difference between hanging in there through the hard times and giving up early on.

Val gave birth six weeks early and little Katie was in the NICU for a month. As a premature baby, Katie did not have the strength or coordination to latch on to the breast, so Val pumped her breasts religiously and provided the staff with a steady supply of mother's milk to nourish her infant. When she finally came home, Katie had mastered drinking from the bottle, but had difficulties with Val's nipples, which were extra-large, about the size of U.S. quarters. Val continued pumping and bottle feeding. She patiently offered Katie her breast regularly for several weeks with no success. She understood that Katie's gestational age was a month and a half younger than her "official" age, and she was still quite tiny. With continuous encouragement from her husband and her doula, she didn't give up, and was rewarded when Katie, at eight weeks of age, opened wide and took the breast into her mouth. From then on they were a nursing couple, with Val feeling very satisfied that her persistence had paid off.

LAID-BACK BREASTFEEDING

We are seeing an exciting new trend in breastfeeding, as mothers are being encouraged to feed their babies in a "laid-back" position, based on the research of midwife Suzanne Colson (2010). The mother takes a comfortable, semi-reclining pose, with her child lying tummy-down across her body. The newborn's cheek rests near the breast, which is continuously available. Mother and baby can be skin-to-skin or the mother can be lightly clothed. Full-body contact encourages reflexive feeding behaviors, and the use of gravity to support the baby makes it easy for him to get the nipple well back in his mouth. Because the mother's arms are free, she can easily guide or assist the infant. Mothers are relaxed and comfortable, and the physiological need of both mother and child for continuity of their connection outside the womb is satisfied. Studies have shown that newborns allowed to rest this way demonstrate significantly increased time in active suckling (Colson et al., 2008).

The concept of Biological Nurturing™, which strives to promote the naturally instinctive behaviors that support successful feeding, includes this style of nursing. As Suzanne Colson, the innovator of this concept says, "the breast is a circle and the baby can approach it from any angle" (Colson, 2009). Mothers and babies can find their own comfortable position, even after a cesarean birth. The goal is comfort and ease with both bodies relaxed. Due to the force of gravity, the milk flow is moderate, allowing more efficient digestion and elimination, and less spitting-up. You can find more information on this approach at www.BiologicalNurturing.com.

POSITIONING THE NURSING PAIR

Mothers may also decide to sit up to breastfeed as they may have been taught in their breastfeeding classes or books. When mothers are in these sitting positions, it's important to help their babies achieve a deep latch by paying attention to positioning. Both mother and baby should be comfortable. Many women like to have a "nursing station" where they know they can nurse easily, and where the things they need are kept close by. It may be a rocker, a spot on the couch, a big cushy chair, or in bed. The baby can be across mom's body, in her arms, or laying prone on her body while the mother is in a comfortable reclined position.

Many mothers enjoy the support of a breastfeeding pillow, which is commercially available in a variety of styles, but these are not always necessary. This pillow, or a firm pillow from around the house, placed on mother's lap, can help bring the newborn to the height of the breast, allowing the mother's arm and shoulder muscles to relax. Place the infant in a belly-to-belly position, facing the breast, so the baby doesn't have to turn his head to suck and swallow. He requires firm head and body support, or he will become anxious and floppy. Newborns must focus fully on sucking to be successful. If the baby is prone on his mother's body, gravity supports the baby, giving him good head control and allowing him to make his way to his mother's breast and latch on.

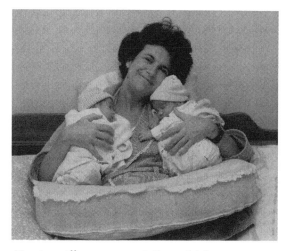

Nursing pillows are especially useful for managing twins —Photo credit: Frederick Yukic

The mother may need help finding the right combination of pillows to create the proper support, or ideas for getting her own body comfortable and relaxed. Often a pillow under her elbow can relieve tense muscles. You may remind her to breathe if she holds her breath in fear of discomfort, tensing her body and sending the wrong signals to both her child and her milk ducts. Relaxing the body is very important for easeful nursing.

Another feeding position is known as the "football hold." The infant's feet are tucked behind the mother's elbow, the back and head are cradled in the hand, and brought to the breast. This is a convenient hold for nursing twins, and there are extra-large nursing pillows to accommodate nursing two at the same time. It can be a useful position to try when there is nipple soreness, as the pressure of the infant's palette will be at a different spot on the nipple. It also allows the baby to approach the breast head-on, which may be easier for some, particularly for mothers who have had cesarean births.

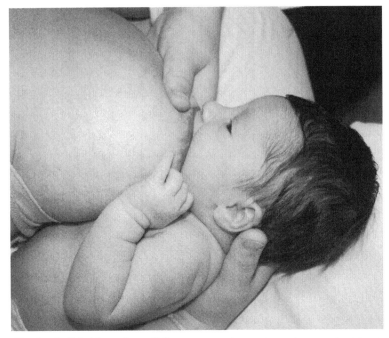

The football hold works well for some nursing pairs —Photo credit: Maggie Muir

Nursing in a lying-down position works for some moms, even in the beginning. The baby's body will need to be well-supported, and he may need the mother's help finding the nipple. This is a restful position for the mother and often is used as the baby gets older and develops more neck strength. The mother lies on her side with one arm under her head. She pulls the baby into her breast with the free hand, belly to belly, and continues to support his head and back as he latches on and begins to suck. A pillow or rolled receiving blanket against the baby's back can help maintain his position. Moms with different body types will find different degrees of success with this position, but generally it can be mastered with the increase in baby's muscular development.

LATCHING ON

The baby should be placed nose or top lip to nipple, encouraging a wide-open mouth, then pulled in close as he latches on, taking in as much of the areola as possible. A "C" or "U" hold around the breast can be helpful if the mother has large breasts or the baby is having trouble latching on. Have the mother think of holding her breast like she would a large sandwich. The direction of the "sandwich" should be in the same direction as the baby's mouth. The mother can guide the nipple into the wide mouth, or tickle the lips to get baby's attention. Gentle kneading of the breast can encourage let-down.

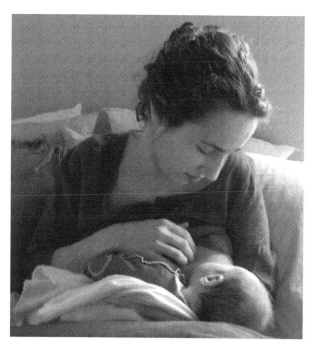

Comfort and relaxed positioning is easily achieved in a cozy bed —Photo credit: Salle Webber

A newborn will find his way to the breast and self-attach to the nipple if placed on his belly, skin-to-skin with his mother in a semi-reclining position. This is a restful way to feed and can be especially valuable if the mother is tense or the infant is struggling.

It is important that the newborn learn to take the nipple well back in his mouth, taking as much of the areola into his mouth as he can. This stimulates the full let-down, assuring him of receiving a complete and satisfying feeding. If the baby is having difficulties, you can help him by gently drawing his chin down as he latches on and begins to suck. It's OK to remove the nipple and begin again if his

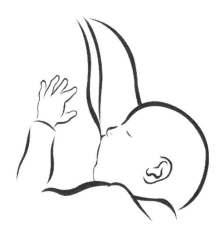

A deep latch can ensure that breastfeeding remains pain free —Illustration credit: Ken Tackett

latch is too shallow. Have the mom slip her finger into the corner of his mouth to break the suction before she removes the baby from her breast. He's developing habits now, so this is the time to insist on a wide-open mouth. Nipple soreness is often the result of a shallow latch, which damages the nipple and leads to incomplete draining of the breast and an unsatisfied infant.

Kelly said, "I feel so sorry for my baby, my milk is pouring too fast into her mouth and she's choking and sputtering. Then she seems to have so much gas! What can I do?"

If the breast is very full and flowing fast, the baby may be overwhelmed with milk. If the breast is engorged and hard to the touch, the baby may have trouble getting a good latch. In either of these situations the mother can prepare for the feeding by manually expressing enough milk to soften the breast; pumping some out for later use; or by taking a warm shower and letting some of the excess milk flow down the drain. A relaxing shower can put a new mom in a perfect mood for a leisurely feeding. Gravity can also help when the baby is prone on the mother's chest; the laid-back breastfeeding position helps slow the flow of milk.

ONE BREAST OR TWO?

There is no rule about whether to nurse on one or two breasts at a feeding. Both approaches have their advantages, and it is up to each nursing mother to decide what works best for her based on her milk production and her baby's feeding patterns and weight gain. Though we recognize that the glands are continually producing milk and never are really empty, it is often recommended to allow a newborn to drain or soften one breast before switching sides. Some newborns only require one breast per feeding. Remember which breast is up next! Moms may often forget. On the other hand, switching sides when baby becomes drowsy can stimulate more intake, as well as increase prolactin[1] secretion in the early days and weeks. Mothers can finish one side completely and offer the second breast. For good breast health, alternate draining is ideal, so start on the less-suckled side for the next feeding. Remember that a newborn's stomach is smaller

[1] Prolactin: a hormone secreted by the pituitary gland that stimulates and sustains milk production.

than her fist, more like the size of a shooter marble, so overfilling may result in spitting up the excess. Sometimes allowing a baby to rest for a while between breasts can increase the amount she consumes with less spitting-up. The caregiver can encourage the mom to take time for a relaxed and patient feeding.

Women also vary in the amount of milk storage capacity they have, based on how much glandular tissue their breasts contain. A mother with a large storage capacity will generally have enough in one breast to complete a full feeding, while a mom with a smaller storage capacity may need to feed from both breasts.

Occasionally an infant will refuse to nurse from one side. One mother previously had a breast biopsy, which caused the spray of milk to go askew in the affected nipple. Neither of her babies would nurse from that side, so she fed entirely with one breast. She felt lop-sided for many months as the milk production in the unused breast ceased, but her body accommodated the infant's needs with just one busy breast. Another mom's son refused a nipple that had a small tag of extra skin, and apparently was uncomfortable in his mouth. This woman pumped her unused breast, keeping it ready for the day when he would accept it, which occurred at about one month of age.

NIPPLE CARE

If the new mother's nipples are feeling tender, it may be because they are delicate and not used to being in a wet mouth for hours each day. They will get used to their new job quickly with proper positioning. Any soreness that exceeds very mild tenderness needs to be investigated by a qualified professional, such as an IBCLC (International Board Certified Lactation Consultant).[2] Most hospitals

[2] To find an IBCLC in your area, check the ILCA.org website.

have certified lactation specialists on staff as well. Sustained painful breastfeeding means that something is amiss, such as a tongue tie in the baby or yeast or other infection in the mother.

Frequently we see a shallow latch, where the baby is sucking on the nipples rather than further back. This will be uncomfortable for the mother and will affect the efficiency of let-down. The mother may need her doula's assistance in evaluating the baby's latch. Observe the nipple as the baby comes off the breast. The latch is problematic if the nipple appears compressed or pinched. Start over, patiently encouraging the wide latch, which will ultimately leave both baby and mother satisfied.

There are various ways to treat sore nipples. Air-drying, leaving breasts exposed as much as possible, or a little sun can help. Ultra-purified lanolin is helpful for moist wound healing and can also help with pain if the mother has cracks or fissures. But lanolin only treats the symptom, minimizing pain while the nipples heal. The cause of the nipple soreness also needs to be investigated and addressed. A shallow latch is often the problem. Sometimes practitioners may give mothers lanolin to treat the symptom of sore nipples without addressing the cause. This is not effective care. Lanolin products don't need to be wiped off before the baby nurses.

Except in cases where thrush is present, expressing a little milk and applying it to the nipples is also very healing, Nature thought of everything. Incidentally, breast milk is also beneficial in the infant's eyes if they're goopy or in the nose if it's stuffy. It's a miracle substance, never duplicated by science. If nipples are feeling tender, snug bras should be avoided. Breast pads can be useful, but need to be changed when they become soggy. A damp breast pad is not helpful when nipples are raw. Mothers can also go braless while at home, or buy a few nursing tanks that offer support and make breastfeeding access easy.

If soreness persists, mother and child should be examined for the presence of thrush or bacterial infection. Thrush is a persistent yeast condition that passes back and forth from baby mouth to nipple. Thrush is addressed more fully in the chapter "Colic, Reflux and Thrush," and should be diagnosed by the healthcare provider.

Signs of bacterial infection include an area of the breast that is red, hot to the touch, or has visible pus. The mother may also report fever or flu-like symptoms. Mothers may have an infection even when they do not have a fever. Any infection should be treated right away, to avoid progression into a more serious problem, such as a breast abscess.

FLAT NIPPLES

Some women have nipples that are flat or inverted, in varying degrees. Frequently, gentle sucking, pumping, or manipulation can coax them out. Then the baby can get a hold on the nipple and draw it out, retraining it over time. If this is difficult, a nipple shield can be used for successful feedings. This is a thin silicone nipple placed over the real one, which the baby sucks on as the milk is released and the mother's nipple is gradually drawn out. One mom's nipples refused to emerge through nursing two children, and she used a nipple shield for every feeding, but it is more common that the nipple will respond and change within a couple of weeks, no longer requiring the shield. A breast shell is another helpful device that is worn between feedings to draw out the nipple. Flat nipples do not impact production or flow, just ease of latch. Tools, such as nipple shields and breast shells, should be used under the supervision of a qualified healthcare provider, such as a lactation consultant. Incorrect or indiscriminant use of these tools may create additional problems over time.

THE SLEEPY NURSER

When Bonnie and Garret brought little Cody home, they were waking him every two hours around the clock, as they had been told by the doctor to do. His birth had been difficult, and his weight dropped a bit too much by his second day. At my visits they expressed their exhaustion at getting up so often. Sometimes he simply refused to wake up to eat, and they fell back into bed frustrated, knowing he would need to be fed in another hour. They took long naps when I was there, keeping up this demanding schedule for two weeks, as Cody grew and slowly became aware of his body. When it was clear he was waking up on his own and gaining weight adequately, they were able to relax and follow his lead. Breastfeeding became a joy, a reunion of mother and child, rather than an anxious chore. When our time together ended at three months, Cody was the biggest child in the mom-and-baby group, a chubby and vigorous feeder. He and Bonnie had become an easygoing, on-demand nursing pair.

Being born is exhausting, and many infants are sleepy for a few days afterward. Weight is carefully monitored, and newborns usually lose five to ten percent of their birth weight in the first few days; more than that can be a cause for concern. Sometimes a newborn must be reminded to eat by being wakened and gently stimulated, particularly a late preterm or under-five pound infant. Rubbing a foot, changing a diaper, or removing a blanket or clothing can bring her back to Earth, as can talking to her, kissing her, stroking her limbs and head, or tickling her mouth with a nipple. She may nurse briefly, then fall back to sleep. If so, arouse her again, burp her, sit her up and say "Hi." Massaging the breast while nursing can help keep her actively sucking by encouraging a steady flow. It can be hard to get a sleepy baby to nurse, but we don't want her to become dehydrated or undernourished. This sleepy period will not usually last more than two weeks and is more common in smaller babies.

The baby's doctor may be insistent on seeing weight gain. At the same time, this is a bit of a grace period for both parents and infant, as they are all in need of extra rest. My recommendation is to be vigilant about feeding your child, at the same time be kind to yourself and continue to trust the natural process. Anxiety is rarely helpful.

A most wonderful way to approach the sleepy baby, or the mom who feels she may be under-producing, is with uninterrupted skin-to-skin contact. Tuck the mother and child into a cozy bed, with nothing but a diaper on the baby and the mom's top uncovered. Allow constant access to the breast. Let the little one lounge on her mother's body. The smell and feel of her mother's skin will arouse the infant to feed more frequently than if she is wrapped in a warm blanket, sleeping in her grandma's arms. Both mother and infant will be stimulated by the other's presence, and a deepening of the connection and bond will also occur. This can be a time, as well, for the depleted body of the mother to enjoy deep rest. The doula can facilitate this by setting up a comfortable space, with mom's food and drink, and maybe a good book, readily accessible. Mother and child should be encouraged to remain this way for at least a full day ... or two. If this is not an option, suggest an hour or two of naked snuggling. Providing the baby with full skin contact at each nursing session is helpful in keeping her active through the feeding.

Permit me to mention the doula's responsibility to support the parents in following through with doctors' instructions, while maintaining the right to offer practical suggestions based on the wisdom of experience, and intimacy with the situation. I remember when my own first son was born, in 1972, the focus in the maternity ward was on getting the babies on a schedule, and regardless of the infants' hunger, they were fed every four hours. As soon as I was home, after the required four days of hospital stay, I began feeding my son on demand.

Today's parents face a medical profession whose emphasis is on weight gain. As the parents are becoming familiar with their newborn and learning to understand his needs, they may be advised to feed him differently than their intuition guides them to do. They may be advised to supplement with formula, to leave baby in the care of nurses, to awaken him frequently, or not to breastfeed at all. They may look to their doula for guidance, even for "permission" to do it their way. We are not medical professionals, and are not in the business of contradicting the doctor. Professionally, it is our responsibility to guide couples to follow sound medical advice. If the advice is not sound, then perhaps it is our responsibility to say so. There is little black or white here, and lots of room for discussion.

Encourage your couples to pay close attention to their child, to get to know what's normal for him or her, and to develop confidence in themselves as caretakers. If they've been advised to wake the baby for feedings, it is prudent to do so, until they feel they can read him better and can monitor his daily intake. They will be reassured by plenty of soiled and wet diapers, and then they can begin to relax and allow him to initiate feedings. This is part of their process as emerging parents, their empowerment as the experts on their own child. Let them find their way as you praise their small victories, and encourage them to recognize how much they already know.

If you find the medical professionals in your area to be poorly educated about the advantages of mothers' milk or how to assist women to nurse, it may be your job to refer moms to lactation consultants, Nursing Mothers' Counsel, La Leche League, Breastfeeding USA, or the Australian Breastfeeding Association for support and information. You may have a few books available to lend on the subject. The accommodating doula will be well-informed and able to offer sound suggestions or referrals.

THE SQUIRMY NURSER

It is not uncommon for an infant to become squirmy and unfocused during a feeding. If there is anything distracting going on in his body, he will not be able to pay attention to the work of sucking. He may be uncomfortable, and as much as he wants that warm sweet milk, it is only adding to his discomfort.

An infant in this state, perhaps kicking his legs, arching his back, thrashing, wailing, pulling off the breast and wanting to go back on, needs to be picked up against the chest or shoulder, or held leaning forward in your lap, and assisted to burp or fart. Or, you may soon see and hear evidence of a bowel movement. When these functions are completed, and pressure is relieved, nursing can begin again. It's a matter of attention. The newborn needs to focus on the act of breastfeeding. It requires coordination: suck, swallow, breathe. If he's trying to poop, his body needs to focus on that; if he has a painful gas bubble moving through his intestinal tract, he will wiggle in discomfort. Keep in mind that all his systems are immature, but he is growing and adapting every day.

A new mother sometimes reads this distressed behavior incorrectly, assuming that the infant is upset because of a lack of milk. She feels she must be responsible for the problem, she must not be providing what the baby needs, when in fact it is his own body he's dealing with. We encourage the new mother to be patient with the infant and trust in herself.

The trend toward laid-back nursing, in a comfortable reclined position with the baby belly-down across the mother's body, may also resolve some of the distress patterns we see in newborns. The help of gravity with baby's digestion and to encourage moderate milk flow, as well as the increased ease with which the newborn can latch deeply can contribute to a comfortably fed infant.

Jocelyn, a slender and small-breasted woman of forty had reservations about her ability to nurse. When Jack would fuss and wiggle at the breast, she assumed she didn't have enough milk. Squirmy sessions often ended with a bottle of formula. When I began coming over to help and observed this fussy behavior, I asked her to take him off the breast and comfort him, patting his back and holding him upright. He let out a big burp! Soon he was able to go back to the breast, calmly. At the next feeding, he began to fidget, she sat him up and within half a minute he pooped. Jocelyn recognized what was going on with Jack, and began to trust that her milk supply was sufficient, and that her body indeed could do its job.

IS THE BABY GETTING ENOUGH?

If there are worries about whether the baby is getting enough to eat, the best barometer is dirty diapers. There should be at least six to eight wet diapers a day after the mother's milk has come in, and many newborns poop in almost every diaper as well. We can teach parents to recognize a sufficiently wet diaper by placing three tablespoons (45 mL) of water in a clean diaper and letting them feel its weight; a sufficient poop is at least the size of a U.S. quarter. Weighing the baby with a highly calibrated scale is another way to assess his intake (these scales are available for mothers to rent. Scales available at baby stores are not accurate enough to assess the baby's intake.) After the initial loss of a few ounces, it is considered normal for a newborn to gain three-quarters of an ounce to one ounce a day, and by two weeks of age or earlier we expect an infant to have regained her birth weight. Lactation specialists sometimes perform a "weigh-feed-weigh" check, where the newborn's breast milk intake in ounces is evaluated. Alerting new parents to the sound of their baby swallowing, like a whispered "k" or "kuh" during feeding, can also reassure them that their baby is nursing well at the breast. Generally, newborns can be observed for signs of normal thriving: sleeping well; nursing vigorously 8 to 12 times a day ending with that content "milk-drunk" baby falling off the breast; wet and soiled diapers; gradually longer periods of alertness between feedings; attentively gazing at mother and father.

PUMPING

The use of a breast pump may be recommended if the infant is hospitalized, when there is concern about sufficiency of milk production, if the infant is unable to latch on, if the mother is returning to work, or if the mother desires to allow someone else to feed the baby. A manual pump may be sufficient for a mother who needs only an occasional bottle, but if the baby is not feeding at the breast, a hospital-grade electric pump may be necessary to generate sufficient milk production. Electric pumps are available in a variety of styles, and are efficient and comfortable to use. Most hospitals offer rental breast pumps.

The body is encouraged to produce more milk by the additional stimulation of the pump, and it can keep the flow going if the baby is unable to suckle. The milk pumped out can be fed to the child with a bottle or other feeding device, or stored for later use. Some fathers decide to offer the baby a bottle once each night, or on weekends, to allow the mother to sleep through a feeding. Bottle feeding of breast milk is also useful to facilitate appointments or a quiet dinner for two. Pumped breast milk can be stored for three or four days in the refrigerator (some say six days, but I think the taste and consistency change by then), or up to six months in the freezer. It is also safe to let it sit at room temperature for several hours (http://www.llli.org/faq/milkstorage.html)

DOES MATERNAL AGE MATTER?

Though some may disagree with me, it has been my observation that older moms, those around forty and up, often need to work a little bit harder than their younger counterparts to provide an abundant milk supply for their newborns. I sometimes say to these women, treat nursing like a full-time job, which it is. You'll be putting in about eight hours a day. Give yourself plenty of rest in between nursing sessions, feed yourself well, and drink plenty of water. Make nursing a priority. For women receptive to "alternative" treatment, acupuncture and Chinese herbs have been shown to be very effective in supporting lactation in the perimenopausal mother. Your body, as the vehicle for the process of milk production, must be well cared for, as it was in pregnancy. As you produced a perfect child, so, too, you can feed him.

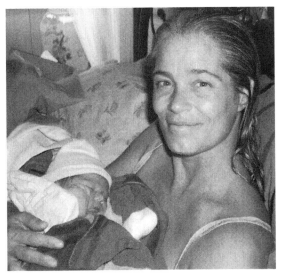

This 44-year-old mom birthed her third son at home and nursed him for over two years —Photo credit: Blaine Michioka

SEEKING HELP

Clara had nursed her first two children and anticipated uneventful feeding of her third. However, the infant couldn't seem to latch on, her rhythm was off, milk went everywhere. Clara pumped her milk to bottle feed, but little Emma couldn't seem to

accomplish this either. Milk ran down her chin and mother and baby were frustrated. A clean eye dropper solved the immediate problem of satisfying her hunger, but the condition persisted. A consultation with a lactation specialist uncovered the issue … immature muscular coordination in the infant's mouth. Time was expected to solve the problem, but meanwhile, the parents relaxed and found other ways, such as the eye dropper and the finger-feeding tube, to nourish their infant with her mother's milk.

In many communities, breastfeeding support is easily available and freely given through The Nursing Mothers Counsel, La Leche League, Breastfeeding USA, or the Australian Breastfeeding Association. These are wonderful organizations with trained counselors available to provide mother-to-mother support for breastfeeding. Sometimes more specialized practitioners, such as lactation consultants, must be called in, if the concern is unusual or difficult to identify. A doula should always feel comfortable suggesting a phone call to one of these experts. Pediatric physical or occupational therapy may be useful for infants with sucking abnormalities. Most often, with determination, patience and guidance, a new mother and baby figure it out and nursing progresses successfully.

THE MIRACLE OF BREAST MILK

When Ramona gave birth to her second child, she made the difficult decision not to breastfeed, though she had contentedly nursed her first baby two years earlier. Somewhere in between, depression had set in, and she had found relief with the use of an antidepressant medication. Her doctor told her that breastfeeding

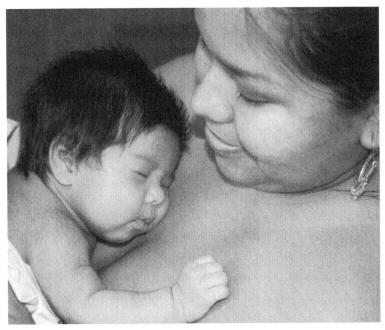

Keeping mom and baby close will encourage physical and emotional bonding as well as successful breastfeeding —Photo credit: Maggie Muir

was contraindicated, and Ramona felt that her state of mind was the more important factor for her baby's well-being.

At three weeks of age, baby Damon was diagnosed with a kidney disorder. His parents gathered many pages of medical reports on this rare condition. It seemed the disorder could be overcome in infancy, but if not, would require a lifetime of dependence on antibiotics. Furthermore, one of the substances that had been shown to facilitate improvement was breast milk!

This was sufficient inspiration for Ramona. It was clearly more depressing to have a sick child than to stop the medication. By now Damon was four weeks old, and Ramona began putting him to the breast. Within three days of his vigorous suckling her milk was flowing and meeting his demand! Joy replaced depression as her child healed fully.[3]

The potency of mother's milk should not be underestimated. Just as the woman's body generates the perfect conditions for development of a fetus, it continues to provide exactly what the infant needs at each stage of growth through breast milk. No commercial product comes even close to the vitality present in fresh mother's milk.

[3] I do not suggest that a woman using an antidepressant cease taking the medication without the careful monitoring by a doctor. Not everyone will fare as well as Ramona. The point of the story is the body's ability to re-lactate after suppression, as well as the power of a mother's love for her child. Additionally, some antidepressant medications are considered compatible with breastfeeding; if a mother wishes to breastfeed, the need for medication may be an obstacle for her. Board-certified lactation consultants (IBCLCs) have resources the mother can take to her physician to discuss the best course of action for her to take. Also, refer mothers to the InfantRisk Center for up-to-date information about medications and breastfeeding: www.InfantRisk.org.

Chapter 17

THE BREASTFED BABY'S FIRST BOTTLE

Jennifer won't be going back to her doctoral program until her breastfeeding son is a year old, but she hopes to allow her husband, mother, and in-laws to feed the baby now and then. She purchased a breast pump and we discussed its use. When I arrived one Monday, she told me that over the weekend her husband Jon had tried to feed baby Eli a bottle, twice, and it had been a complete failure both times. On further discussion, it seemed they had decided to try the bottle after he breastfed, because they didn't want to annoy him while he was hungry. Mom stayed out of sight in the other room, while dad called out play-by-play commentary. Someone had told them not to force the bottle on him, but to offer it. So Jon, also a graduate student, expressed a drop of milk onto the tip of the nipple and held it a half-inch from Eli's lips, waiting for him to take it voluntarily. He didn't.

I laughed heartily at this news. Fortunately, these parents know that I love them. I explained that, first of all, he has to be fed a bottle when he's hungry, otherwise, what interest does he have? Next, if mom is in the house, and dad is speaking to her, though she's not answering, Eli is aware of her even without visual contact. Close the bedroom door, take a walk, or sit outside in the yard. The bottle should be given without the mother's presence.

And most importantly, put the nipple into his mouth! It's a foreign object to him; he has to learn its value and purpose. He may resist, but sliding the nipple over his tongue, gently, not

forcibly, stimulates the sucking reflex on the palette. Coax him.
I offered to try to feed Eli a bottle, and Jennifer agreed. After
lunch, she pumped about two and a half ounces from her breasts,
and went off for a short walk on a beautiful, clear day. I asked
her to give us twenty-five or thirty minutes. Eli had begun to
squirm, and within five minutes of her departure he was giving
hunger signals. I sat down and positioned us both comfortably. I
approached Eli's mouth with the bottle, inserted it, and he began
to suck! No fussing, no resisting. A fast learner! That was one of
the easiest first bottles I have ever given. He drank for a while,
pulled off, and burped on my shoulder. Back to the bottle, he fin-
ished it gracefully, and was fast asleep when his mother returned.
Because she had pumped just before the feeding, they were still in
sync and she would be ready when he was. We laughed together
at all the lessons babies have to teach us, regardless of our level
of formal education!

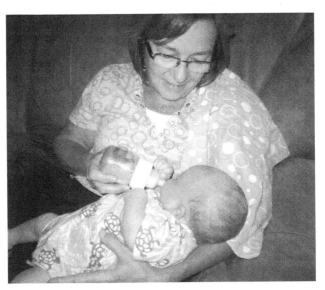

The breastfed infant is gently introduced to the artificial
nipple —Photo credit: Sarah Bennett MacLeod

It is generally agreed that a window of opportunity exists for successfully introducing a bottle of expressed breast milk to the baby. Around four weeks is often considered the optimum age, as the baby is strong and experienced at sucking, while still young enough to be agreeable to a new way of eating. Certainly many babies accept the bottle earlier or later. Anytime can be the right time, depending on the circumstances and the need for the mother to be away from the baby. But in a flexible situation, I suggest trying it around four to five weeks, and ideally by an experienced person, and then keeping it up a couple of times a week for "practice."

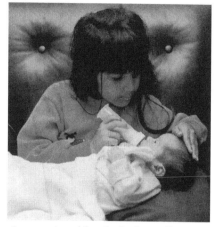

An occasional bottle-feeding allows other family members to participate in nourishing the baby —Photo credit: Fatima Kazimi

At five weeks postpartum, Dustin's mommy asked me to help her prepare and set up the breast pump a friend had loaned her. She purchased the individual-use parts that touch the body and the milk, and we got the machine ready to go.[1]

---

[1]Please note that most pumps on the market are not designed to be multi-user devices, even when the parts that touch the milk are changed. If the motor system is not a closed system, contamination can occur. A fairly expensive and sturdy item, many women do share their pumps.

Three days later she had pumped four ounces, was feeling very satisfied, and eager to offer Dustin a bottle. Her husband suggested I feed and he watch the first time. I showed him how, if the breast milk has been chilled, to gently heat the bottle in a mug of hot tap water, swishing it to mix and warm the milk. Holding Dustin at a nice upward angle, with good head support and eye contact, a burp cloth under his chin, I tickled his lips with the nipple, and inserted it into his mouth. He played with the nipple with his tongue, pulled it in and pushed it out, took a few random sucks. Then he stopped, had a big poop, and relaxed. I changed Dustin's diaper and returned him to feeding position, where he readily took the bottle, figuring it out almost immediately. His dad was impressed! Dustin seemed quite content. After almost fifteen minutes of sucking, he took a break, and we saw that he had consumed one ounce of breast milk. That, too, surprised his dad, who thought it was much more. In another ten minutes he consumed another ounce and a half, and then was clearly finished.

The newborn-size nipple worked great—no leaking out of the sides of his mouth, no heavy gulping, and no frustration. It is very important to have a nipple with a small hole and slow-flow, designed specifically for newborns.[2] I gave Dustin several opportunities to burp during the feeding, and small breaks. His mother was out of the room when he woke up and throughout the feeding. In most cases, the baby will resist receiving a bottle from his mother, from whom he expects to receive the breast. This is the job for someone else, so

[2]For more information on finding a bottle that works for a particular infant, go to www.breastandbottlefeeding.com/.

that Mom can get a few extra hours of sleep, go to an appointment or out to dinner, or work outside of the home.

Some babies are not as readily agreeable to the artificial nipple as Dustin or Eli. Squeezing some milk onto his lips or tongue can get the baby's attention, and interest him in trying the bottle. It is important to be persistent—gentle, but persistent. It's an entirely new concept for the child. As I was beginning to feed Dustin, I was calmly telling him that he was learning something new about life; that people besides his mother can feed and nurture him.

If, however, he absolutely refuses, appears angry and very resistant, then certainly back off. Perhaps this is not the right moment for him. Try again later. You may notice shortly that he'll have a bowel movement or a burp. This could have been distracting him and making him uncomfortable. Babies need to be focused to eat. It's a job requiring coordination and attention. I have known babies who never accepted a bottle, but in most cases they were offered the first bottle significantly later than four weeks of age.

A young dad recently told me, "I'm glad you said to be persistent, because I had to be, and it worked. I think I would have given up because at first Zachary really seemed annoyed to have the bottle put in his mouth." He expressed a few drops of milk on his baby's lips. Soon Zachary was sucking happily, and his dad felt successful, and now able to nurture his son in a new way.

Chapter 18

COLIC, REFLUX, AND THRUSH

COLIC

In normal circumstances, babies are not always entirely happy. One of the most common postpartum issues is what we call colic. If the child cries regularly, inconsolably, for two or more hours a day, generally in the evening, we say he is colicky. The condition can go on for weeks, and is frequently outgrown by four months. The word colic is derived from the Greek word for pain; but some researchers believe the condition to be one of over-stimulation, and say the brain waves of colicky infants look more like anger than pain. Probably the reasons for colic are varied, including both gastrointestinal discomfort, and the need to release tension taken into the body from excess stimulation.

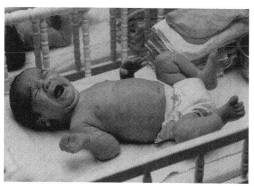

The call for comfort —Photo credit: Leila Kazimi

Newborns have immature neurological systems, and some are more sensitive than others to bright lights, lots of people, noise, and the like. It is wise to maintain a calm environment for the newborn, especially if he appears to be disturbed by sudden noises, a visit to the supermarket, the company of active children, or someone talking to his mother while he nurses. If he exhibits colicky behavior, lessening stimulation may help him: dim lights, swaddling, and white noise. Breastfeeding or a pacifier can help him pull himself together, providing the dependable rhythm of the suck, lessening his internal chaos. If this behavior occurs regularly for several days, parents of colicky babies are wise to prepare themselves for the expected bout of crying by eating and getting comfortable before the usual fussy time begins. Often by swaddling or bundling the baby in advance, and beginning a period of quiet rocking or walking, we can help to lessen the severity of the upset. Wearing the baby reduces crying and encourages rest, and is most comfortable for the adult.

Another culprit in the evening crying challenge may be overfeeding. This can be tricky to recognize. Sometimes a mother's tendency is to offer the breast at every whimper. By evening, the little belly may be so full as to be uncomfortable. And what is the loving mother's response to her baby's cry? She offers the breast again, thus compounding the problem of discomfort. Babies do love to suckle, but may not need the extra fluid. An over-full infant will pull on and off, thrashing and complaining, often spitting up abundantly. This is where a pacifier or a clean finger can be very useful. Wrap the infant snugly against your chest, with a pacifier in place, and move gently up and down and side to side. Or step outside and walk around if weather permits. Keep the child very close and contained, so she's not thrashing. Tune in and help her find her comfort zone. Do what works. Hum, chant, sing lullabies. Inhale and exhale deeply. She will feel your breath and begin to relax. If she burps, farts, or poops, you may try feeding again if she seems to be more comfortable and still wakeful.

There are also times when what the infant seems to want is to be put down. This usually comes as a surprise after all other efforts have failed!

REFLUX

Gastroesophageal reflux occurs in many healthy babies, being a result of an immature digestive system. The esophageal sphincter muscle opens and closes to allow the passage of food into the stomach. If this muscle becomes relaxed, it may allow a backup of milk mixed with stomach acids, causing vomiting and a burning sensation in the throat. Spitting up is common in infants, but for some it is so extreme as to be considered a disease. These babies exhibit frequent and projectile vomiting, often seeming to lose everything they've taken in, failing to gain weight as a result. Some infants exhibit silent reflux, not spitting up but crying hard, often after a burp. In both cases, they require being held upright for at least a half hour after each feeding, and do best sleeping at an upward angle. Babies with reflux often cry significantly more than others, appearing to be in pain. We know that the throat becomes raw and burned by the acid backup. This may cause the child to resist feeding at all, or sometimes the opposite: there seems to be comfort in the sucking. Feedings should be small and frequent, and ideally in a calm environment. It is best to elevate the baby's head while feeding, and to gently help the baby to burp often, keeping air bubbles from building up in the stomach.

Let gravity help to keep the food down, by holding the baby

upright and not jostling, and design a way to put the child to sleep at an angle, either by elevating one end of the cradle or bassinet, or creating a nest with firm pillows, in which the head is elevated. Many parents find themselves sleeping with the baby upright against their chest, certainly the baby's preferred spot! Unfortunately, the parent rarely sleeps soundly in this position. A Tucker Wedge can provide a comfortable and safe sleeping area for the child with severe reflux.

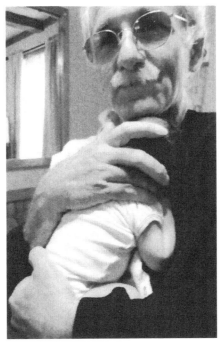

Grandpa's patience soothes the infant into rest —Photo credit: Karen Rowe

In some cases, medication to decrease gas or neutralize stomach acid is prescribed, with varying degrees of success. The bottom line is time: most babies outgrow reflux by six months to a year. In my experience, reflux runs in families. The babies I've seen with severe acid reflux have older siblings who also suffered the ailment. Parents of these children come up with solutions, like swaddling and swaying, white noise, a walk outdoors, taking turns caring for the crying infant and enlisting support from relatives. I emphasize that many babies experience frequent, uneventful spitting up, but in a few cases it is severe enough to warrant extra care and lifestyle solutions, as well as possible use of prescription medication.

June's fourth baby had reflux, just like all the rest. Her first child had been afflicted for a full year. June thought her baby would never be happy! The second, her only boy, threw up a lot but was never as miserable as the first. The third and fourth both required being held upright long after each feeding for about the first four months of life. June even invented an angled cushion upon which to change diapers. If the baby began to vomit, she wouldn't stop until she was empty, so it was important to carefully and calmly hold her upright after feedings. June and her husband spent long hours walking the halls in the middle of the night. Somewhere during her third baby's early months she discovered the power of "white noise." If her daughter became inconsolable, standing near the stove and turning on the fan became an almost foolproof way to calm her. It also worked for baby number four.

THRUSH

Thrush is a condition that can affect baby's mouth and diaper area, as well as mother's nipples. It is caused by an overgrowth of the yeast *Candida albicans*, which is present in the normal digestive system. Babies also pick up yeast as they travel through the birth canal, but the use of antibiotics, which remove beneficial flora in child or mother may encourage a proliferation of these natural inhabitants. The immature immune system of the infant may also allow this imbalance to occur.

The presence of white patches on the tongue, palette, or inside the cheeks is the primary symptom of thrush, but be careful not to mistake leftover milk residues for those pesky spots. The white patches of thrush will resemble cottage cheese, but can't be wiped away. Mother's irritated nipples, not healing normally but becoming increasingly sore and uncomfortable, and a spotty-red diaper rash on the baby are other signs of possible thrush. This is an irritant to the digestive tract, and can cause fussiness, soothed by sucking, although some babies will become very unwilling eaters, causing another concern. This condition is most common where there have been antibiotics taken by either mother or baby, but is not restricted to these situations, and is not a rare condition.

Often the nursing mother afflicted with thrush will complain of deep pain, under her areola, or pain that lingers after the feeding is through. The nipples may be inflamed, with a pink or red sheen or a flaky appearance. Normal nipple discomfort is resolved with improving the latch. Nipple problems caused by thrush often begin after the initial adjustment to nursing is over, when instead of progressive ease, the mother finds herself in increasing discomfort.

The doctor will prescribe an anti-fungal ointment to apply topically, and perhaps a medicine for the infant to take orally. It has also been seen that a diluted vinegar or grapefruit seed extract solution swabbed on affected areas can clear up the problem. When my son was small, the accepted treatment was a diluted solution of gentian violet, which worked but was a bit messy with its deep-blue stain. The style of treatment will depend on the severity of the problem, and the parents' orientation to treatment options. In my experience, it can be an annoying, uncomfortable, and persistent problem, making early detection of thrush most beneficial. If I think I'm seeing it in a baby or mother, I will discuss the condition, and recommend having it checked by the medical practitioner.

If pacifiers or bottles are being used, it is important to clean the nipples and pacifiers in very hot water between uses, to prevent reinfection. This is also true of pump parts, breast pads, bras, towels, or anything else that touches mother's nipples or baby's mouth—wash after use in the hottest water possible. Mother's nipples can be gently rinsed and air-dried. We encourage exposure to air as much as possible for the nipples of nursing mothers, and most especially when the condition of thrush is present. Swabbing with a mild vinegar solution between feedings can help disinfect the nipples. Use a mixture of one teaspoon apple cider or white vinegar to one cup warm water. This alters the pH of the nipple and discourages yeast growth. The discomfort of nursing on painful nipples is disruptive to the enjoyment and success of breastfeeding. As the comfort and well-being of our mothers and babies is our concern, we want to be aware and educated about the possibility of thrush.

SECTION III

THE BUSINESS OF CARE

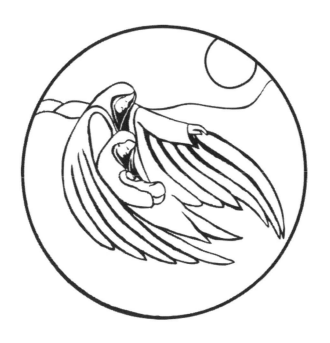

Chapter 19

THE ART OF BUSINESS

If working as a postpartum doula is your goal, you must decide what style of doula you will be. You might prefer to work through an agency; in a team of two or more doulas; or on your own. How much experience you have, your level of confidence, your temperament, and your lifestyle are important considerations. How are other women in your area working? Call and ask them. Doulas are by nature receptive and sharing people, and will help you get started.

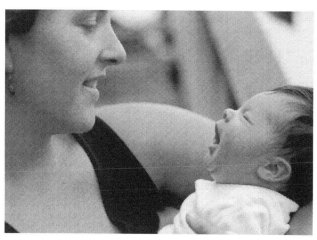

Why we do what we do —Photo credit: Ed Sale

WORKING ARRANGEMENTS

Working for an Agency

In some metropolitan areas of the country, postpartum care service agencies are providing families with the help they need after a birth. Caregivers are trained by the agency's staff and matched with families who have requested the services of a doula. The client pays the agency's fee for service, out of which the doula is paid an hourly rate, and the company collects the balance. In these situations, the doula herself does not make contracts, financial agreements or procedural decisions, but leaves these things up to her employer, the service agency. Advertising and client screening is taken care of, and the doula works where she is assigned. In large cities, working with an agency may be the preferred option for parents who have no other way of checking references of a potential caregiver. They are assured, as well, that she has been trained for this job. The doula receives direction, ongoing education, and experience.

Owners of these service agencies determine whether their doulas will be employees or sub-contractors, and how income will be reported for tax purposes. They design manuals of expected behaviors and techniques, and provide training sessions for their doulas. Regardless of the particular details of each agency, the work of carefully tending the new family remains the same. The doula is ultimately a reflection of her own unique sensibilities and temperament. Your work will speak for itself as you gain experience.

Working Independently

If you prefer to work as a doula in private practice, you must develop your own organizational plan to handle the business end of the profession. There are decisions to make about hourly fees, minimum hours, contracts, and prenatal meetings. A phone number must be provided, and brochures or business cards are necessary. You must consider your availability, and how many families you can serve at once. The geographic area is another consideration—how far are you willing to travel for a client? Decisions must be made about exactly what you do and do not do in service to families. My friend Cathy was a great doula, but her idea of "dinner" was a pot of brown rice. She clearly told families before they hired her that she didn't include cooking in her service.

Working as a Team

Two or three doulas may organize a team approach, sharing clients and backing each other up in case of a sick child, unexpected family needs, or personal illness. Potential clients will want to meet all of the doulas in advance, and are reassured that there will always be someone to care for them. In some cases, these teams provide both labor and postpartum support.

The Case for Simplicity

As a practicing doula, it has been my intention to keep things simple. I use my home phone for my doula service. That way the expense is minimized, and when I'm not home, my gentle husband, one of my daughters, or perhaps a grandchild will take a message or let the caller know when I might be in. I keep it small and personal; postpartum is no time for formality. Email is another great option for easy communication.

I charge a flat hourly rate, and offer a free prenatal visit. I have no written contract, only a verbal agreement with the parents, after our meeting, that it is their intention to engage me as their doula, and my intention to be available to them. I ask that they give me as much information as they have about their needs, such as hours per day, days per week, how many weeks, preferred time of day, etc., while recognizing the multiple unknowns inherent in birth and postpartum. I strive to be as flexible as possible, understanding that they can only guess at what their needs will ultimately be.

A More Business-like Approach

Other doulas may choose to be more businesslike than I am. A telephone line designated only for your business, with a professional-sounding message, may be your style. You may want to require a signed contract, stipulating a minimum number of hours of service or a specific schedule. A deposit may be requested to hold your time. You may offer a package, such as 15 hours a week for two weeks, for a certain price. Your business can be as loose or as structured as you want. It is your business.

You might also design a card, flier, brochure, or website to advertise your work. How you will express yourself here requires careful consideration. Lovely artwork or touching photographs can enhance your presentation of your skills and offerings.

Set Priorities

I prioritize families, generally, in the order in which they engage my services. If I have a family that expects to want afternoon help, any other family that contacts me for the same time period will be informed that my afternoons are spoken for, but if morning help would be useful for them, we can talk further. Clear communication on my part is essential to keeping expectations at a level that can be easily met. It is challenging, but I trust that I will be directed where I need to be in each moment. Once, I was expecting to help two moms who were due four weeks apart. One woman anticipated needing only two weeks of support. She, however, gave birth two weeks past her due date, while the other woman, expecting her third child and wanting lots of help, gave birth two weeks early. Both babies were born on the same day! To meet the needs of both families, I worked two fifty-hour weeks. It was demanding, but temporary. My own family pitched in to help at home through my extra-busy workdays, and both postpartum families were cared for.

One of the beauties of this work is its ever-changing nature. No two weeks are ever alike. A demanding or tiring situation will soon be a memory. If we find ourselves overbooked, we learn to be more conservative in making commitments. Finding balance is an ongoing issue. We want to help everyone we can, but if we disappoint them by not keeping our commitment to be available, we are no help at all.

Be Clear About Your Availability

It is essential to be clear about your availability. If you have children that need to be picked up from school, a job, weekly class, meeting, or other commitments that present time restraints, be sure to be clear with your potential clients about these. You do not want to generate expectations that you cannot meet. Nor do you want to deprive your family of the care they deserve, or yourself of the things in your life that are necessary and nourishing.

How flexible we can be may parallel how effective we can be for our postpartum families. I strive to be open to schedule changes, cancellations, and extensions. Frequently, a friend or relative comes to stay for a few days, and she can assist the new mom, rather than me. This is reasonable. I recognize that it may be a financial strain to hire a doula, and the family should be the first line of support. I am with them as a backup, to cover when they cannot.

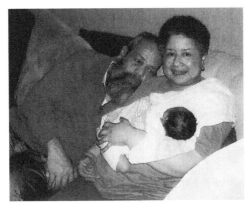

Family members can be the best caregivers, but aren't always available —Photo credit: Christina Mann

On the other hand, if a doula depends on a certain income, she can establish a contract stipulating the number of hours per week she will assist, and how many weeks of service she will provide. How formal we wish to be is up to each individual caregiver. I have found that what a family expects to need and what they ultimately do require can vary greatly in either direction. A contract can protect a doula who has reserved her hours for a specific family.

What to Charge

Setting your fee requires looking into the local prevailing wage charged by others doing similar work, considering what is appropriate for your level of experience and what feels sufficient for the service you provide. You may not want to price yourself out of the range of moderate-income families, though there may be plenty of upper-income clients available. This is a personal choice. I have raised my rates several times because younger and less-experienced doulas were charging more than I was! It is my choice what I want to earn, and I give myself a raise when it feels like the right time. I am also open to reducing my fee or doing a partial trade for a family in need of support with limited funds. Each doula must consider her position on this. I recommend being open to doing some "community service" as a way to practice giving of yourself without financial return, building your experience base, and serving your world by caring for those in need of the skills you have.

Being a volunteer postpartum caregiver can provide excellent experience and training, while offering service to someone who might not otherwise receive support. It is an honor to be allowed into the sacred space of new life, and humility is an appropriate attitude.

Gift Certificates

Postpartum care is a wonderful baby shower gift, or a present from grandparents or other family or friends. Many people would like to assist a new family, but don't know how or aren't available themselves. Paying for doula care is a great option. Often, the request for donations to pay the doula was made with an invitation to a shower or blessingway (a ceremonial preparation for birth) when I was a parent at the Santa Cruz Waldorf School, where I had the honor of serving a number of families in this role. It's a great way for the community to support its members. Organizers of baby showers are in the perfect position to suggest pooling funds to hire a caregiver. As the doula, you may have a gift certificate available, and suggest this gift idea on your brochure.

Andrea's grandfather wanted to help her with her new baby, but he knew his skills were limited. When a friend told him about postpartum doulas, he called together Andrea's several uncles, and collected donations to hire a doula to assist her. His generosity was noted by a family friend, who added her donation. Andrea would have been on her own those first weeks, but because of their thoughtfulness on her behalf, she had naps, meals prepared, baby and household care, and someone to model the new skills she needed to learn.

Minimum Hours Per Visit

You may want to establish a minimum number of hours per visit, especially if your geographical range is large. I have set a minimum of two hours, though I recommend that, if possible, families have doula care for at least three or four hours per visit. We can accomplish a lot in that time: shower, nap, lunch, conversation, household maintenance, and baby care. But each situation is different, and we must be flexible to meet the circumstances. I tell a client, "This is about getting your needs met. This is not about me. Tell me what you need." I do my best to meet those needs within the allotted time frame. Some families' budgets may allow only two hours a day of help. In these households, I work quickly to accomplish as much as possible in a short time, wanting to ease the burden of the new parents. One mom who used her savings to pay my fee, said, "This is the best money I ever spent."

Getting Paid

I keep a record of my hours and present the parents with a statement, a pre-printed invoice with my logo, date, time, and hours, which I fill in, each week or two. We cannot expect new parents to keep track of our hours. Now and then, I see a very organized mom who knows exactly what she owes me and has the check written, but more often, the mother of a newborn exists in a timeless bubble. When I want to be paid, I simply ask, "Would you like to write me a check today?"

The Initial Contact

When potential clients first contact me, I determine if I expect to be available at their time of need, and if they live within my geographical range. If so, I answer their questions about my service, and give a general overview of what a doula can do for the family. I ask if there are other children and what they expect to need. If they wish to proceed, I offer to make a free prenatal visit at their home, for an hour or so, ideally when the whole family can be present. Meanwhile, I mail or email them my brochure and a copy of an article I wrote about my work. I ask them to read it, and then call to set up a visit. In some cases, they are ready to make an appointment at the time of the initial phone call.

Home Visit

Visiting the family in their home gives them an opportunity to interact with me in their personal setting, and I can view them in their natural surroundings. This is the time for them to ask any questions at all, about my experience or my philosophy of childrearing, my willingness to do household tasks or errands, and to get a feeling for me as a person they might decide to invite into their home. I explain my focus on rest, nourishment, care of the whole family. I let them know I am a mother and grandmother. If they have children, usually watching me from a safe distance, I smile at them often and include them in my conversation. I am willing to be interrupted by a small child's desire to show and tell, realizing that this child's opinion of me is highly relevant, and we will become good friends if I am warm and open. I may ask what the parents want from a doula, and what other assistance they may receive. We discuss practical matters, such as my fee, their preferred hours of care, anticipated need for food preparation, or housekeeping tasks they want attended to.

This is my opportunity to express any limitations I may have regarding the work I do. I make it clear that I am not medically trained. I might have very specific availability at their time of need. If I plan to be out of town at any time that may be important to them, I am sure to let them know. If it feels that we are a potential "match," I may ask for a brief tour of the house, discussing food preferences as we see the kitchen, and sleeping arrangements in the bedrooms. We might talk about what kind of diapers they plan to use (cloth, diaper service, or disposables), and if they have the basic baby necessities.

Some parents ask my advice about what to purchase or how to set up their baby area, and this is a way for us to get to know each other. They see that I am easy-going and not interested in having every latest thing being marketed for babies, but I do know what the essentials are. They hear my philosophy that a baby needs the loving arms of its parents, milk and warmth, and a few diapers. The rest is for our convenience. I let them know that their comfort and harmony are my highest priorities, and that I will be open and flexible to meet their needs. Flexibility is the key word here. Prenatal parents do not know for sure how things will go for them. Hard labor? C-section? High-needs baby? Unexpected complications? They are taking a leap of faith, and I take it with them as I agree to be there beside them when the time comes.

How we present ourselves at this initial meeting will make a big impact on the potential client. How we will relate to their newborn and other children is vitally important to these parents. We will be in their home at a delicate and vulnerable time. They must feel safe with their doula; they must trust that she has their best interest at heart and is gentle and wise. I encourage each doula to consider her personal philosophy and how she might express it. Be true to yourself and true to your clients.

> *You came to meet me seven or eight months pregnant, with a willingness to just hang out until I was comfortable. You answered so many questions for me just by being yourself and sharing life experiences you have had with previous clients. It impressed me that you never boasted about how many babies and parents you had actually cared for. But clearly, your mannerisms and sense of self told me, "This woman knows."*
>
> —Lisa, mother of two girls

After all has been said, I ask the couple to discuss their needs and give me a call when they have decided if they want me to save my time for them. Sometimes they already know, and we verbalize an agreement on the spot. Otherwise, I await their call.

What if a doula interviews with a family she doesn't want to work for? This happens to me rarely, but when it does, I encourage the parents to look for another helper. I may express time or distance limitations, or in other gentle ways explain my lack of availability. If it's not a match, probably the clients will feel it, too, and keep looking.

However, I am happy to work with people who have different beliefs and behaviors from my own, if I feel I can be of use. I learn much from my clients with different lifestyles, and we have a great experience together. I caution potential doulas against being too rigid in their selectivity. At the same time, we must refrain from martyrdom, and say "no" when it feels in our best interest.

Checklist for the Prenatal Interview
The Birth
What is the due date?
Who is the midwife or doctor?
Where is the birth expected to be?
Taking birth preparation classes?
Are there any special circumstances?
The Emerging Family
Is this the first baby?
If not, what are the names and ages of the children?
What are their schedules and needs?
How can the doula best help them?
How much will the father or partner be available and for how long?
Will there be support from other relatives or friends?
Details
Will the mother be breastfeeding?
Have feeding stations been set up?
Do they anticipate needed help with nursing?
What type of diapers will be used?
Is there an organized area for diaper changing and dressing?
Do they need help with this?
Where will the baby sleep at night?
During the day?
What are the family's food needs and preferences?
Will friends be bringing meals?
How much food preparation can the doula help with?
What are the eating routines of the children?
What housekeeping tasks will the family need help with?

A tour of the house is appropriate.
Are there pets in the home?
Will the doula help with them?
How about plants and gardens?
Will there be a need for errand and shopping assistance?
How many hours per day and days per week will doula care be desired and for how many weeks?
Is a specific schedule of care required, or is there flexibility in scheduling?
Delicate Areas
What are the expected emotional needs?
Are there fears that we can address?
What do the parents hope for by hiring a doula?
What have previous postpartum experiences been like?
Is there anything else the family wants the doula to be aware of?

Preparing Yourself for the Day's Work

The personal presentation of the doula is important. We arrive at the home appearing rested and refreshed, clean, with teeth brushed. Clothing should be simple, casual, soft, attractive, colorful but not loud, and fully washable. The infant will be resting against the doula's chest, so tops should be free of buttons or zippers. When I work in more than one home in a day, I bring along an extra shirt to wear for the second family. I may have spit-up or other bodily fluids from the first baby on my shirt, and I want to provide a clean area for each infant to rest. Makeup is unnecessary, and the scent may be irritating to baby or mother. No perfumes, for the same reason.

The doula should eat before arriving at the home, and may want to carry her own snacks or lunch. Many families will ask the doula to help herself to any food in the kitchen, and this is appreciated. I will sometimes eat a piece of fruit, or a few bites of vegetables as I prepare lunch. A slice of cheese or some crackers, an energy bar, or a handful of nuts can keep my energy up. Often there are leftovers that I might sample, but I try not to spend much time eating when I'm working. My time in each home is limited, and I want to accomplish as much as possible.

With intention, the doula leaves her own worries outside the door. We don't spend time talking about our problems; instead we are present to help this family with their needs. Meditating first is an excellent practice (see Meditation Before Entering the Home of a Newborn, Appendix A, for a recommendation). Some moms will ask about the doula's family, and express genuine interest. In sharing our lives, we acknowledge the growing friendship with the postpartum family. At the same time, we don't use valuable time chatting about things that have no relevance to the situation at hand. This is a matter of balance, and the doula must maintain awareness of her role as both friend and paid caregiver.

Upon arriving, the doula should wash her hands thoroughly, before greeting the baby. Hands must be washed after changing a diaper, using the toilet, touching the family dog, or handling the trash.

Know Your Boundaries

I used to joke that the only household task I was unwilling to do for my families was to clean up dog poop. Then, while working with a beloved family who had three small dogs in the house, I faced that boundary and was forced to remove it. The eldest of the dogs, old Clarence, had an "accident" on the floor at the foot of the stairs. His owner was at a doctor's appointment. I was at home with baby Connie. And the dogs. Clearly this mess couldn't wait for Mama Sandy to return home, so I laughed at myself, tucked Connie into her bassinet, and set about cleaning

the disgusting pile. I am, as I often say, a professional mother.
And what mother could leave dog poop on the floor of her home?

A doula may be limited not only by preferences, but by her physical condition, age, beliefs, or other responsibilities. There are lines each of us is unwilling to cross, and we must respect ourselves. For example, some doulas have a "no sickness" policy, and will not come to the home if there is an ill family member. An older doula may prefer not to work with families with active toddlers. Being asked to clean the kitty litter box or walk the dog may be too distasteful a chore for some women. It's fine to say "no, that's not in my job description."

I personally have found very few things the postpartum family needs done that I can't or won't do. Taking the garbage out is no big deal. Staying an extra half hour on a challenging afternoon is fine. Going out for groceries or to pick a child up from kindergarten is what's most needed some days. If I iron a shirt for her husband's business meeting, the new mother won't have to stand at the ironing board herself. It's my job to serve. It's easy to figure out how to do that, if I am willing to see the work of the home as holy work, sacred and good and necessary.

Yet all this must be done within the bounds of self-honoring and self-care. I do not accommodate requests for heavy lifting or moving furniture, and no longer give piggy-back rides to four year-olds. The caregiver must respect her own body and heart, maintaining her energy in order to give it back many-fold to those she serves.

We must consider our personal boundaries. What tasks will we limit ourselves to? Will we clean the toilet? Walk the dog? Take out the trash? Drive the toddler to daycare? Will we drive a client and her baby and kids in her car to a doctor's appointment? Will we massage her feet or scrub blood out of the sheets?

I have said yes to all these things, and many more. My philosophy is that I am another mother in the house. I do what mothers do, which is just about everything. Clients are generally respectful and more than reasonable. Issues of liability can be serious, so it is advisable to give some thought to driving for clients. Some doulas have liability insurance for their practice. These are individual decisions, and I suggest looking into the prevailing mode of the region where you live and work, as well as your personal inclination in these areas of responsibility.

GETTING STARTED

A business card or brochure is very helpful when introducing yourself to the community in which you want to work. A brochure allows you to explain the role of a doula, and to offer some information about your background and experience. A business card should clearly identify your profession, and offer contact information. Artwork or photography can add a personal and meaningful touch.

With your carefully designed card or brochure, stop by the offices of local midwives, OB/GYNs, and pediatricians. Introduce yourself to the staff working at the desk and tell them what you do. Ask where you might leave some of your cards. Check with local hospitals for prenatal classes, and call the women who are teaching these classes. They are the ones who regularly see the pregnant women, and they may be interested in mentioning your service in their classes, making your brochures available, or recommending you to couples who express an interest in postpartum support. Perhaps they might invite you to speak to a class, explaining your service. The local lactation specialists in the hospitals and private practice, and those who volunteer with La Leche League, the Nursing Mothers' Counsel, Breastfeeding USA, and WIC, all work with newly postpartum women. Let them know you are available, and reciprocate by suggesting their classes, services, and offerings to families you meet. It is great to have some references, families you've helped or who know you well who can speak for your professionalism and abilities. Once you get started, the momentum picks up as your name gets known in your local birth community.

COMBINING SERVICE WITH BUSINESS

We do this work because we love it and also because we need to earn a living. We go joyously to our jobs, and that in itself is a gift to the families we serve. Yet we are paid, and that separates us from the casual friend or family member offering to help out. It gives the new mom permission to ask us to do chores she may be reluctant to ask of others. As well, we have no emotional "baggage" in relation to the family and no long-term agenda. The nature of our work is intimate, informal, and personal, yet professional. The mother may see us as her best friend for several weeks, but in fact we receive compensation for our loyalty, and we will leave her when the time comes. Maintaining this relationship comfortably can be tricky, but with practice it becomes quite natural and functional. Mothers have expressed feeling a great deal of freedom and satisfaction with the personal service of the doula, able to discuss anything with her, from diaper rash to her philosophy of parenting, marriage, and family.

If you work as an independent doula, your practice will be purely a reflection of yourself. Each of us has our own style, personality, strengths and weaknesses. Your reputation will develop over time, as your local birthing community becomes familiar with your work. Although there exist private training and certifying organizations, such as CAPPA (Childbirth and Postpartum Professional Association) and DONA International[1], at present there are no government licensing requirements for postpartum caregivers. We are on our own, and therefore responsible for working with integrity and commitment, upholding the highest standards of our profession.

[1] DONA used to stand for Doulas of North America. As members joined from outside the U.S. and Canada, the name was changed to DONA International.

Chapter 20

TIMING OF CARE

I limit my postpartum caregiving period to the first three months of the child's life. This is the most fragile time for both baby and mother. Certainly the need for support lasts well beyond three months, but then it's appropriate for the nanny, mother's helper, or babysitter to step in. Not only has the child progressed, but the mom has regained her power and no longer requires the protection and care of the initial postpartum weeks. She's usually ready by this time to resume charge of her home and family, and often, it happens earlier. My goal is to be with her to this point, to work myself out of a job.

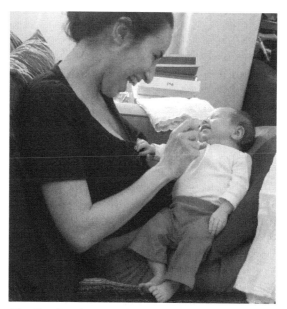

The first laugh is a milestone —Photo credit: Salle Webber

I feel I have succeeded in my work when a new mother begins explaining to me what's going on with the baby, in a knowing voice; when I find her already showered and fed early in the morning; when I arrive and she's dressed and ready to go out, handing me the baby at the door. It is my goal to see her regain her strength and develop a working system for her life in its new form. As she discovers ways to accomplish her daily routines, she is empowered and develops confidence in her ability to be a good mother. At this point, I can safely kiss her goodbye, knowing she's prepared for this phase of her life.

Let me add that, as in all aspects of this work, there are exceptions. For example, one family I helped had a baby girl born six weeks early. She was hospitalized for two weeks, after which I began going to assist in their home daily. My assistance was greatly appreciated by these new parents, both over 40, struggling to care for this tiny one who required pumped milk and bottle-feeding, around the clock, for many weeks. I stayed with them for a full six weeks extra, reasoning that she deserved to be treated like someone her gestational age; that was who she truly was.

In another case, an active home-business family that I got along with beautifully asked me to consider coming over when I had time between newborns, after the initial three months were over. Since I was well integrated into their routines and children's needs, I continued to help out for a few hours once or twice a week for a couple of months. Many years later, I still receive loving notes at Christmas and Mother's Day from this family.

Often, however, I work with a family for perhaps six or eight weeks. Occasionally, it may be only two or three. Each situation is entirely individual. There may be other family members lined up for certain periods, or financial considerations that limit the hours I spend with them. One grandmother gave her daughter enough money for one hundred hours of doula care, and it was up to the new mom to use it as she wished. Another couple had saved carefully to provide themselves with assistance for the first two weeks. A young mother's relatives pooled donations to buy her some help, and then collected a second time when they saw how much she valued the support.

A natural progression often occurs, in which the number of days per week of doula care declines gradually after the first several weeks, tapering off until the work of the doula has been completed.

We know that it takes about six weeks for the mother's body to heal fully after childbirth. In cases of surgical birth, it may take significantly longer. I encourage mothers to refrain from taking back all the responsibilities of home and family care until their bodies are internally healed. This is an investment in their personal health future.

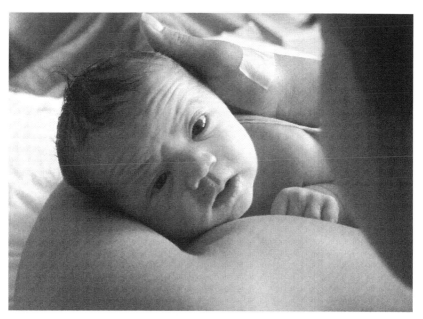

The vulnerable newborn will become a strong, capable baby in a matter of months —Photo credit: Maggie Muir

Ultimately it may be the doula who must gently disengage from the family when the time is right. The mother's level of health and well-being both physically and emotionally are key factors in determining when the doula's work is done. The sense of routine returning to the home, household chores being accomplished without outside help, the mother's focus beginning to expand to include friends and out-of-home experiences—these are the signs of readiness. Of course, a family friend is well-poised to stay on in a helpful role indefinitely. That's what friends do. Those who are professional doulas, however, may want to remain available for the next newborn, and thus are not free to stay with a postpartum family beyond the early months. The separation may be sadly sweet, but remember that this represents the great progress the family has achieved. It is helpful to go back in memory to the very first days when all was new and tender, and invite the new parents to look at how far they and their infant have come. I tell my families that I will always be their doula, and they can call me anytime. And many of them do.

Chapter 21

THE ART OF BEING A DOULA

Postpartum doula care is more an art than a science. This work is not for everyone, and is not a get-rich-quick job. But if it is your calling, you will see this work as vital, honest, worthy, a way to bring deep expressions of caring to the world, one family at a time

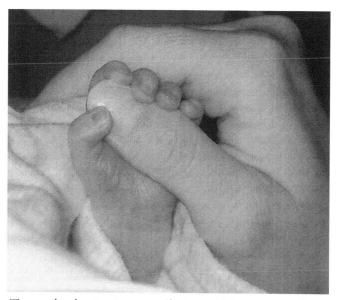

This tender duo inspires our affection and desire to care for their needs —Photo credit: Bradley Brown

BEING OF SERVICE

The art of being a doula includes the art of paying attention and noticing where you can serve. The ability to be of service has to already be an integral part of who you are. If not, you must begin there. Being a mother, of course, is the best training. When a woman first becomes a mother, she is brought to her knees; she is humbled, tested, burned in the hot fires of love. Her self-centeredness, a healthy thing in a growing organism, is transformed, by necessity, into self-sacrifice for the good of her child. It becomes second nature. At first, the ego may fight and squirm in tremendous discomfort. As doulas, we remember this state from our own initiation into motherhood, and are able to compassionately witness the same transformation in the families we serve. Our new moms need our understanding of how unsettling this rite of passage can be. Her life has been changed forever.

> *One new mother, a single woman, came home from the hospital with an unhealed c-section, barely able to lift her baby. Her finances were meager, and her vehicle worn out. She was new in town and short on friends. Her world turned upside down with the birth of her son. Suddenly everything seemed impossible and her self-pity soared. As her doula, I did my best to make her feel comfortable and cared for, to support her in making connections to her new community, to help her find solutions to small practical problems. I reduced my fee for her, and extended my hours. I listened to her sorrows, joys, and dreams, as she gradually healed, gained strength, fell deeply in love with her son, and moved more fully into her new role.*
>
> *My job included washing her dishes, changing her sheets, and helping her jump-start her car; holding the baby while the mother cried in a long, hot shower, and holding her—the new mother—afterward. We brainstormed how to make the house safe for a quickly growing infant, where she could find quality, affordable childcare when she went back to work, and the useful community services that might be available to her.*

As her doula, it was necessary for me to be flexible and intuitive, as her needs were many and varied. This is the daily reality of the doula…tuning in and going with what's happening. We have no agenda of our own but to serve.

CALMING THE INFANT AND THE ATMOSPHERE

The art of infant-holding, the ability to quickly calm the child, is of great value in the postpartum home. How to do the baby dance, that delicate balance of rhythm and bounce, to feel the child's need and to respond, the ability to ease the baby's crying, soothe her to sleep, these are the arts of the doula. Motherhood itself is what usually teaches these essential skills. We learn over time to understand and to respond successfully. It is a tremendous gift to new parents for the doula to pick up their crying infant and lovingly, easily, soothe it into rest. It shows them that it can be done, and it eases their tension in the moment. A crying baby so fully changes the atmosphere in a room, and I'm often amazed at the immediacy of quiet when the little one is held. Such a basic need, being close to another human being; so easy to fulfill!

Catherine had a newborn, a two-year-old, and a home business—lots going on. I did many things to keep the household running smoothly, but what she most dearly remembers, and shares in her annual Christmas card, is the hours I spent holding her infant son. She says she is sure that his sweet disposition and easygoing nature are partly a result of those precious early hours he was held in calm and loving arms.

I have often been told that my calm nature enhances my ability to be helpful in postpartum homes. Babies are erratic and do unexpected things. You never know when a newborn will awaken and demand immediate care. The baby is easily soothed by a relaxed pair of arms, a moderate heartbeat, and an easygoing presence. As the doula, it is not your baby, and you will be going away in a few hours. You are there briefly and for the express purpose of supporting the family with your vitality and loving presence. It is an easy formula for success. You fall in love with the baby, with the mom, with the entire family, yet in a detached way, allowing you to easily move on to the next family when the time is right; but when you are present in their home, just love them. Your purity of purpose will guide you to know what to do in each moment. Allow yourself to breathe deeply and fully, to remain mindful of your function. You are a vehicle of kindness, a source of compassion and understanding. This is a fine role to play, one that will uplift you as well as those you serve.

I find that my personal problems often solve themselves as I devote my attention and care to the new family. Before I enter a postpartum home, I intentionally leave my own concerns and worries outside; inside, another full and real-life drama is going on. I choose to immerse myself in that for a few hours, and frequently, my own concerns rearrange themselves into a more pleasing configuration while I'm otherwise occupied.

MOTHERING THE MOTHER

My primary focus is on the mother. She is the rock upon which her family stands. Her physical and emotional stability are vital, and I can help. I support her in napping and resting by holding the baby and tending the children. I fix meals and snacks, keep her water glass full and close by. I boil up the sitz bath herbs and have them ready when she is. I'm available to listen and reflect as she shares her feelings about the birth and the immense changes she is going through. Since the new mother has just performed the ultimate miracle of delivering forth a child, it is my function to serve and care for her needs, as she carefully feeds and nurtures this precious infant, and as her own body heals and strengthens.

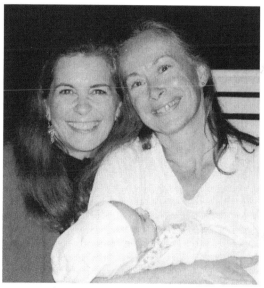

New mothers thrive when they are encircled by a caring community —Photo credit: Jill A. Esteras

Sometimes there is no one else to whom she can safely vent her frustrations, but I empathize, I nod and understand, and perhaps find a way for her to laugh about it. There is a delicate balance between taking her worries seriously and seeing the humor in them. Helping mom to lighten up can be very beneficial, and her trust in her doula is the first step. I can't emphasize enough the need for the doula to radiate an aura of loving confidence and competence, allowing the mother to breathe a deep sigh of relief. Indeed, relief has arrived. A mother of two once told me, "nothing bad ever happens when you're here." I consider us a two-mother household, able to easily handle any little crises that might arise, enjoying ourselves and the children, and sharing together in the flow of daily life—a kind of tribal thinking. I want to leave her with the knowledge that mothering can be fun!

CONSCIENTIOUS HOME CARE

Mothers feel a lot of responsibility for the maintenance of the home, and are often unable to relax when things are a mess around them. I make it a point to scan each room visually, and pick things up as I chat with mom or interact with the children. Dishes and cups left around, socks and shoes discarded by the couch, toys and books strewn about, abandoned tissues and spit-up cloths all can be put in proper places to create a visually-soothing environment. Fluff the couch pillows, fold the blankets, and straighten the piles of books and magazines on the coffee table. It doesn't take long, but produces a very good effect. Sweeping floors is also helpful, pulling together the look of order. The point is, these small things need to be done to maintain the level of comfort in the home, but it is not the new mother who should be doing them.

Doulas aren't generally expected to do "heavy" housecleaning, but definitely should take responsibility for daily maintenance. Pay attention to what is important to the family. Often I ask the parents what household tasks they want tended to daily. One woman told me she couldn't stand a dirty kitchen floor, and she was uncomfortable asking her mother-in-law to mop the floor when she came to help. I assured her that she could comfortably ask me to mop the floor. In fact, I would be paying attention to the cleanliness level of that very floor. The main thing I want to prevent is this newly postpartum mother mopping the floor herself. There are more important uses for her energy right now. I may be the only person in her world that clearly understands that, and is dedicated to being in service to her needs. That is a tremendous gift, and we doulas receive abundant appreciation in return for our devotion.

Let me emphasize the need to be respectful and low-key in tidying up. Don't throw away anything but the most obvious junk. Receipts, notes, envelopes, drawings, can all be neatly piled for future consideration. Really funky refrigerator items can be quietly discarded, but if in doubt, leave it or ask about it. Do not be overzealous, or you will generate another kind of anxiety for the parents. Don't put questionable objects in the dryer or dishwasher. Find the right moment to ask the questions you need answered to comfortably perform your duties. It will ease the mother's mind to know you are paying attention, taking seriously her household concerns, and doing things as she would do them. I repeat, do things as she would do them. This is the Golden Rule.

SENSITIVITY TO THE NEEDS OF FAMILY MEMBERS

If there are older children in the family, it is an art to befriend and nurture them. We tune in to what they really need as they go through their own process of accepting a new sibling. Ideally, the doula will become a welcomed friend, offering food, play, conversation, walks, books, visits to the park, or help cleaning their room. Whatever the circumstances, the postpartum mother will rest easily if she is confident that her children are being tended lovingly and competently.

> *Beth, resting with her third baby, spoke of her five-year-old daughter. "It was such a pleasure, drifting off to sleep, hearing Chloe chattering away, and you responding as you washed the dishes. When I woke up an hour later, I could hear Chloe still talking away, and you still patiently responding. It has been hard to give her the attention she needs since the birth, and I'm relieved that you can do that." I remember that home, and the wonderful, fanciful conversations in which Chloe shared with me her dreams of becoming a midwife and a mother, repeating delightful bits of what she overheard and reminding me where we acquire our values. Chloe trailed around the house with me, chatting busily as I folded laundry, swept, and tidied. She was entirely happy, and it provided great relief to her mom, who valued her naps and baby-bonding time.*

> *When Lillian was a few weeks postpartum, I bundled her newborn onto my chest, put the dog on the leash, and walked with the four- and six-year-olds down the country road to play along the riverbank. This allowed the mother of three to sleep in a perfectly quiet house, in the middle of the day—a rare treat! Not even her husband had the willingness to manage all three children at once. I still run into her now and then, 14 years later, and she always greets me with such gratitude!*

I share these examples to illustrate the qualities of confidence, competence and sensitivity that are so beneficial in postpartum homes.

When the parents know they can trust their doula's knowledge and sincerity in family care matters, it is a huge relief.

There are other people to consider and interact with, too. The husband or partner, as well as relatives and close friends, are much more intimate with the household than you are as the doula. We defer to them, and offer to assist in whatever way is needed.

New fathers are often overtired and anxious, requiring care themselves. I frequently encourage a new dad to use some of the time I'm in the home to get outside, exercise, see a friend, and do something for himself. A nap with his wife may be just the respite he needs, or to have lunch made and served to him, with compassionate acknowledgment of the changes he's going through. Demonstrating baby-care techniques may be helpful to increase his confidence and ability to participate successfully. I'm available for conversation, sharing information, or simple listening, and as a partner in the care of his family. We are a team.

On occasion, new moms have told me that they are counting on me to provide what they know their moms or sisters or mates, however well-meaning, won't recognize or understand. Sometimes, they want support in affirming baby-care practices that their own parent doesn't agree with, such as homebirth, the family bed, or breastfeeding openly. This is tricky. I absolutely want to project love and respect to the grandparents and others, while warmly validating the new parents' choices. No arguments, no judgments, simply creating the space for joyful acceptance of the decisions of the new mom and dad. Laughter is a great tool in tense spots. Also, the doula can share stories of other families she's known. Several times I have witnessed transformation in the grandparents, as they see how happy a breastfed, well-held, tenderly accommodated infant, sleeping in its parents' bed, or nearby, can be. One grandma whispered to me, "I wish I'd held my babies more."

We must take great care to refrain from being a know-it-all. Instead we must delicately offer suggestions and share experiences, and most of all, show by our example that we know what needs to be done, and that we can do it quietly and efficiently. We definitely want the trust and appreciation of the extended family while we honor the new mother's need for our unwavering support of her needs and feelings. This may not always be straightforward, as there can be extended family members who want to control situations inappropriately: a mother-in-law whispering to her son about the unkempt condition of the house or the indecency of exposing a breast in the living room; a persistent older sister who firmly believes in letting the baby "cry it out"; family pressure to circumcise (or not), give a particular name, or attend a family function before the new parents feel ready. There are many areas where a young couple may feel pressured to conform to a style of parenting that is not theirs. A good solution in these cases is to enlist a doula, and part of that doula's responsibility is to stand by the new parents and protect their interests. This is a very delicate dance. We do our best to be compassionate and without judgment at all times, knowing that everyone means well.

We are all on the same side; we all desire the well-being of the new family. Simple explanations and open discussion can often bridge the gap. Again, excellent baby-holding skills will gain the respect of everyone. When that fussy baby is passed to you, and she quiets and soon falls asleep, your talents will be noticed, the value of your service understood, and your opinions requested.

In most cases, family and friends are well-meaning and supportive, though not always aware of what a postpartum family needs. They look to me for ideas of how best to help, and are grateful to know that I'm there when they can't be. I affirm, however I can, that we are a caregiving team, all working together. I often say that I'm the backup person to the real doula: the mother's mother!

FINAL WORDS

The art of being a doula lies in a compassionate and nurturing heart, a willingness to serve others, love of family life and babies, and a healthy respect for the work of the home. If I find myself looking disagreeably at a bathtub that needs cleaning before new mom uses it, I bring myself back to recalling my purpose: to serve the highest good of this woman and her family. This is holy work. We are laying the foundation of this family's life with this precious new addition. We can help to bring harmony, calm, humor, and rest. Our gentle presence can promote general household well-being, as everyone feels that some of their needs have been acknowledged and met, and they can face another day, another night, with this precious and awesome new being. The art of the doula is in flowing, feeling the energy and recognizing where you can serve at each moment. This can be learned and perfected with practice and intention, if one is temperamentally inclined toward quiet service.

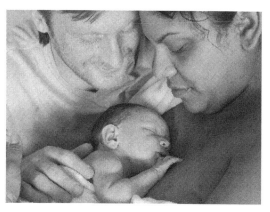

The miracle of life —Photo credit: Maggie Muir

I encourage every postpartum care provider to consider what it is she wants to model. I believe the experiences of infancy are vitally important in the development of the deeply held mental structures with which we respond to life. As more human beings come to see life as good, as filled with loving-kindness, and to see others as friends, more peace will descend on the world. If an infant finds that his calls are not met, that he is left alone with his discomfort; experiences cold, hunger, and lack; is not always treated with respect by others; he may develop a sense of separation, of needing to grasp what he can, of general distrust, or a lack of self-love. As we demonstrate relaxed and contented behavior, we impart these feelings to the child as well. How better to serve the future of humanity?

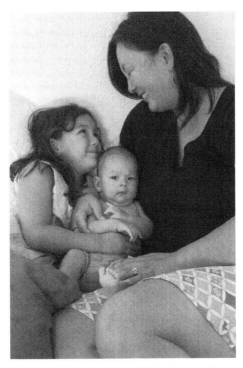

Having been well cared for, this family is now ready to face the world —Photo credit: Maggie Muir

REFERENCES

Colson, S. (2008). (DVD). *Biological Nurturing: Laid-back breastfeeding*. Available from www.BiologicalNurturing.com.

Colson, S. (2010). *An introduction to Biological Nurturing: New angles on breastfeeding*. Amarillo, TX: Hale Publishing.

Colson, S., DeRooy, L., & Hawdon, J. (2003). Biological Nurturing increases duration of breastfeeding for a vulnerable cohort. *MIDIRS Midwifery Digest, 13*(1), 92-97.

Eiger, M., & Olds, S. (1999). *Complete book of breastfeeding, Third edition*. New York: Bantam.

Huggins, K. (2005). *Nursing mother's companion, Revised edition*. Boston: Harvard Common Press.

Kendall-Tackett, K.A. (2007). A new paradigm for depression in new mothers. The central role of inflammation and how breastfeeding and anti-inflammatory treatments protect maternal mental health. *International Breastfeeding Journal*, 2:6 (http://www.internationalbreastfeedingjournal.com/content/2/1/6).

Kennell, J., Klaus, M., McGrath, S., Robertson, S., & Hinkley, C. (1991). Continuous emotional support during labor in a U.S. hospital. *Journal of the American Medical Association, 265*(17): 2197-2201.

McKenna, J. J., & McDade, T. W. (2005). Why babies should never sleep alone: A review of the co-sleeping controversy in relation to SIDS, bedsharing, and breastfeeding. *Paediatric Respiratory Reviews, 6*, 134-152.

Appendix A

Visualize Your Ideal Mother Figure

To inspire your confidence in your ability to be a great doula, it is helpful to call upon the highest form of feminine energy that you can imagine. You are part of this energy that flows through generation after generation of women, and you can access it.

Imagine a female form that represents to you the most perfect example of motherhood. Perhaps she is a spiritual figure, such as Mother Mary or Quan Yin; she may be the Earth Mother or Gaia, or a composite of women you have known or admired in your lifetime. Visualize this beautiful being in your mind, with all her nurturing and compassionate qualities. Allow her to become your connection to the great body of female wisdom, your companion and helper in your work as caregiver.

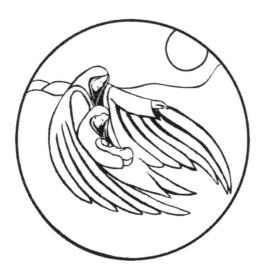

Appendix B

Meditation Before Entering the Home of the Newborn

Sit quietly for a few moments, breathing slowly and with awareness. (In your parked car is a perfect spot for this.) Calm your mental chatter.

Bring your attention to the place just above your head.

Visualize above you, sitting peacefully, the image of the Divine Mother, the pure feminine mother spirit as she looks to you on a very personal level. Feel her presence.

Thank her for her loving guidance. Ask her to fill you today, now, with purity of purpose.

Ask that her wisdom come through your words and actions.

Ask that you may be a vehicle of her compassion and loving kindness, and that all you say and do will be toward the highest good of the family you are about to join.

Feel the strength of your intention to serve, and her joy and acceptance of you.

Allow her to pour her light in through the top of your head, brilliant golden light entering you and saturating your body.

Receive this gift and know you are divinely guided.

Made in the USA
Charleston, SC
23 January 2013